THE **LIFE**
WELLNESS
C O L L E C T I V E™

THE LIFE WELLNESS COLLECTIVE

Faith, Freedom &
The Power of Shared Health

Dr. David M. Shearer, MD & Dorothy M. Shearer, MS, RN

THE LIFE WELLNESS COLLECTIVE

Faith, Freedom & The Power of Shared Health

Dr. David M. Shearer, MD & Dorothy M. Shearer, MS, RN

Copyright © 2026

Dr. David M. Shearer, MD & Dorothy M. Shearer, MS, RN

ISBN: 978-1-968149-08-6

Joint Venture Publishing

The Millionaire Mentor, Inc

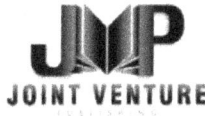

JOINT VENTURE

DEDICATION

To my husband, mother and my father, "Daddilama"—whose unwavering faith, gentle strength, and boundless love continue to guide and support me every step of the way.

To my endearing wife, family, friends, and all who have inspired me—your love, belief, and encouragement have carried me farther than you "know".

We so appreciate all who have cared enough to engage with us—with love, wise counsel, and thanksgiving—offering direction when we needed it most.

Thank you. This book is for you.

TABLE OF CONTENTS

DEDICATION

DISCLAIMER

INTRODUCTION

FOREWORD BY GREG REID

"CHALLENGE BY ADVENTURE"

The Life Wellness Collective "DISCLAIMER"

This book references CareXchange, a Life Wellness Collective operating as a Health Cost Sharing Ministry and Benevolence Access Organization—not an insurance company. Participation is based on shared spiritual beliefs and voluntary support, and CareXchange is not a substitute for insurance and does not guarantee payment of medical expenses. Review all materials and state-specific requirements before joining to ensure it fits your needs.

This book is for general informational and educational purposes only. It is not intended as medical, clinical and/or holistic advice, diagnosis or treatment and should not be used as a substitute for consultation with a qualified healthcare professional. Reading this book does not create a physician/nurse-patient or any other professional relationship with the authors.

Readers are strongly encouraged to consult with their own physician or qualified healthcare provider regarding any medical questions, conditions, or treatment decisions. Do not disregard professional medical advice or delay seeking it because of material presented here. If you believe you may be experiencing a medical emergency, call 911 (or your local emergency number) immediately.

Foreword by Greg Reid
"THE LIFE WELLNESS COLLECTIVE"

There are moments in life that permanently divide your timeline—before and after. For me, that moment came on a day I will never forget, when I received the kind of phone call that every parent dreads: my son Colt had been struck by a vehicle while riding his e-bike. In an instant, my vibrant, joyful 12-year-old boy was fighting for his life—and I was powerless to change it. As a parent, there is no greater agony than watching your child suffer, and no deeper desperation than realizing you can't fix it. I would have gladly taken his place, but all I could do was pray, hope, and act. And that's exactly what I did—I reached out to the people I trust most, the tribe I've built over years through my journey in personal growth and development.

Among the first I called were Dr. David Shearer and Dorothy Shearer, RN—two extraordinary humans who've dedicated their lives to healing, not just through conventional medicine, but through a truly integrative and holistic approach to wellness. They didn't hesitate. They stepped in with unwavering calm, clarity and conviction. Their wisdom and guidance became a lifeline—not only for my son, but for me, and Colt's Mom.

What unfolded over the following days and weeks was nothing short of miraculous. While the hospital followed its protocols, David and Dorothy brought insights and interventions that challenged traditional norms—but they worked. From nutritional support and energy-based modalities to emotional resilience practices, we witnessed subtle shifts that gave us hope. And with each new day, my son showed signs of a comeback that exceeded all expectations.

This book, The Life Wellness Collective, written by the very people who stood with us in our darkest hour, is more than a guide— it's a gift. It's a collection of knowledge, heart, and practical wisdom from two of the most compassionate and brilliant minds I know. Their work is grounded, accessible, and deeply human. It challenges the status quo not for the sake of rebellion, but for the sake of better outcomes—and that's exactly what they helped us achieve.

I believe with everything in me that David and Dorothy helped save my son's life. And in doing so, they helped save mine too. If you're holding this book, you're holding more than pages of advice and information--you're holding a roadmap to true wellness. The Life Wellness Collective is a reminder that health cost sharing truly is health caring. Read it with an open mind and an open heart. Because when the Shearer's speak, we would all do well to listen.

Sincerely,

Greg Reid

INTRODUCTION

Health is never meant to be a solitary pursuit. From the beginning of time, communities have gathered to care for one another, sharing knowledge, resources, and compassion to ensure that no one walks the journey of healing alone. It is this spirit of unity and support that lies at the heart of this book. We are so excited that you are taking the first step in reading The Life Wellness Collective which describes issues with current healthcare, and presents a holistic approach to healthy solutions utilizing health cost sharing as a community to pay for medical expenses, availing more freedom and choices. After all, there are plenty of examples and data that show the benefits of an integrated and functional approach based on health outcomes, and not the checklist of an insurer. Finances and health touch every human being and seeking council versus opinion often makes the difference between wealth (affluence) and well-being. Science has a long way to go before understanding the everyday miracles of the human body. Ethics and medicine should not discriminate, and patient advocacy is necessary to maneuver a complex health system.

As a physician and nurse team, we have witnessed firsthand both the remarkable advancements of modern medicine and the limitations that can leave patients feeling overwhelmed, isolated and financially burdened. Our decades of experience have led us to seek out approaches that not only address illness but also nurture wholeness, community, and faith. That is why we are deeply passionate about the concept of health cost sharing, and equally about the sharing of knowledge, wisdom, and encouragement that empowers people to live well.

The practice of health cost sharing has deep historical roots, within faith-based communities, where participants pooled resources to cover one another's medical needs. This was more than a financial arrangement; it was a way of life. It represented solidarity, compassion, and a recognition that the well-being of one is connected to the well-being of all. In many ways, this model of community care reflects the same principles that guide our own philosophy: with an integrative, holistic, and grounded approach, we wholeheartedly believe that healing is strongest when it is shared.

As a dynamic duo—doctor and nurse, partners in both life and calling—we have long believed that healthcare should extend beyond prescription and procedures. It should be about connection. About choosing whole, natural foods. About preventing illness through intentional living, education, and empowerment. About bringing faith and compassion into every interaction. In this book, we bring those values together with the principles of health cost sharing, offering a vision that is both practical and deeply human.

Our hope is that these pages will inspire you to see health not just as an individual responsibility, but as a collective journey. To consider the ways we can share—not only in the costs of medical care, but in the wisdom, practices, and encouragement that sustain true wellness.

We invite you to walk with us through this exploration of health cost sharing, both in its practical benefits and in its spiritual and communal richness. May it empower you, uplift you, and remind you that in caring for one another, we find the truest form of healing. Enjoy the read and we've also added a bit of an adventure along the way?

Healthy Regards,

Dorothy and David

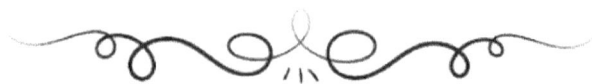

Challenge by Adventure
Unlock the 'Life Wellness Secret':

Within these pages you will find yourself being transformed into a new level of awareness and transformation. In order to make things interesting, we've created a little challenge! Let's engage in climbing the "Transformational Life Wellness Pyramid" together with a theme that involves transitioning from personal health to collective empowerment. You will transcend the pyramid achieving 6 levels of proficiency. Within these chapters, you'll find a health concept in the form of a question, which leads to uncovering a mystery word which, when combined, contributes to the final phrase — the Life Wellness Secret — and maps a step in the journey from awareness to action. Each question will be identified by a key (🔑). Can you find all of them and experience the 'Life Wellness Secret Unlocked?' We know you can do it so let's get started and enjoy the journey!

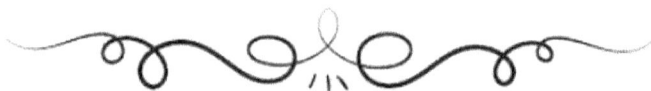

NOW ENTERING LEVEL 1:

Awareness & Foundation

CHAPTER 1:

"A WAKE UP CALL"

The healthcare system is broken and has proven to be a devastating problem. Since when did it become acceptable for chemically-based pharmaceuticals to dominate over nutrition, while substituting artificial solutions over natural God-given remedies only to result in the tragedy of a population poisoned with side effects? Since when does access to care have to be an issue? Since when does one walk into a doctor's office, where questions about mental health are hurled unnecessarily, only to result in yet another prescription medication? Patients are being forced into allopathic healthcare without holistic/complementary choices, and this trend surprisingly continues today in a day and age when alternative and integrative medicine has proven to be a great option. How did this happen?

Let's take a step back in time and look at some very interesting and historical facts whereby John D. Rockefeller, during the early 20th century, changed the face of healthcare forever. While some may take this to the point of conspiracy, realize that at that time he controlled the largest oil company in the U.S.A. known as Standard Oil Company which created a huge net worth equaling approximately 500 billion dollars in today's money. In 1911, Standard Oil was split into 34 separate companies secondary to a Supreme Court ruling that the company had become too large of a monopoly.

This contributed even more money to J.D.R. Following the vast accumulation of wealth, J.D.R. donated $100 million to a philanthropic initiative in the form of a "General Education Board," with the concept to establish common rules and guidance within hospitals and medical schools across America. The slogan became "A pill for an ill." In 1913, he founded the Rockefeller Foundation and together with the prestigious Andrew Carnegie, J.D.R. placed Abraham Flexner in charge of visiting all the medical schools and hospitals in order to establish the leading 100. This resulted in the Flexner Report, which further recommended centralizing schooling and emphasizing and adopting the "germ theory." From here, the pharmaceutical archetype selfishly targeted and matched specific germs to be treated with certain drugs. Healthy living, diet, nutrition, exercise, and hydration were all left by the curbside!

Rockefeller then financed an initiative to streamline and consolidate new programs and adopt the concept of a growing pharmaceutical industry. As a result, approximately 50% of medical schools were forced to close their doors, and some physicians were even jailed for continuing to practice homeopathic, osteopathic, nutritional and integrative therapies. As the Rockefeller Foundation continued its growth, it funded more than 50% for the League of National Health Organization to which its central philosophies and structure still exist today in the World Health Organization.

Now combine this with the Pure Food and Drug Act, founded by Dr. Harvey Wiley, and signed into law by Theodore Roosevelt in 1906. Dr. Harvey Wiley was the Director of the Bureau of Chemistry which was established in 1901 as a successor to the U.S. Department of Agriculture's Division of Chemistry. The funding and establishment of the Bureau of Chemistry can be traced back to the Agricultural Appropriation Act of 1901 (31 Stat. 930), which re-designated the Division of Chemistry as the Bureau of Chemistry effective July 1, 1901. At the same time, there is an evolution of pharma involving Monsanto in Missouri as a chemical company, founded by John Francis Queeny, who financed the firm with his own money and capital from a soft drink distributor, to produce food additives such as the artificial sweetener saccharin, caffeine, and eventually aspirin, too. Who else is known for aspirin? Bayer, who created the first tablet-form aspirin which appeared approximately in 1900 and became available without a prescription in 1915, making it the first synthetic, over-the-counter, mass-marketed medicine around the world. Aspirin became a household name and part of American culture with the popular slogan: "Take two aspirin, and call me in the morning."

Is this all a coincidence? Now let's combine this with the evolution of healthcare insurance as we know it today. Dating back to the 1920's, there was no insurance per se, rather there were industrial sickness funds and prepaid funds within industries that provided healthcare coverage to workers and their families. The Great Depression led to massive unemployment, as well as financial insecurity and instability, making it impossible to afford healthcare. In order to provide some assistance, employers began offering health insurance as a benefit to allure and entice workers. In 1938 the American Medical Association (A.M.A.) agreed to support health insurance, leading to the development of Blue Cross and Blue Shield plans which changed the landscape of healthcare forever, while expanding the reach of the pharmaceutical industry. During World War II, job opportunities were scarce, coupled with unfair and challenging wages, spurring employers to compete for workers by offering health insurance as a benefit.

Insurance as we know it today, was further shaped by labor union negotiations for better benefit packages, government policies and regulations such as Medicare, Medicaid, the emergence of H.M.O. 's, P.P.O.'s, and most recently, the Affordable Care Act. However, tying insurance to employment made things more challenging for those who became unemployed, switched jobs, or became disabled. Furthermore, healthcare providers were enticed by the "fee-for-service" model as more procedures and services increased revenue, leading to quantity over quality, and further contributing to rising healthcare costs.

In 1992, the U.S. Congress passed the Prescription Drug User Fee Act (PDUFA), allowing industry to fund the U.S. Food and Drug Administration (F.D.A.) directly through "user fees" intended to support the cost of swiftly reviewing drug applications. With the act, the F.D.A. moved from a fully taxpayer-funded entity to one supplemented by industry money. Net P.D.U.F.A. fees collected have increased 30- fold—from around $29 million in 1993 to $884 million in 2016. Is this transition working? Moreover, Medicare Part D's new out-of-pocket cap is changing patient behavior and forcing patients, providers and payers to adapt to a 27% spike in drug spending. Yet, based on data on the latest United States Population Division, the U.S. is approximately number 48 on the list of nations for life expectancy at 78+ years of age, behind Panama and Albania. Let that resonate for a moment and consider regions like Asia, Italy, Sweden, and Denmark (just to name a few) live 3-6 years longer (Avendana & Kawachi, 2015). And why are there Blue Zone regions of the world where people are consistently living to 100+? Why does this dichotomy exist and what has to happen in the current healthcare system to regain our health? We have a moral obligation and responsibility to consider healthcare options and alternatives. We would be remorseful if we did not mention artificial intelligence (AI), in this book.

Over the next decade, artificial intelligence (AI) will likely transform medicine by enhancing diagnostic accuracy, personalizing treatment plans, and improving operational efficiency. AI-powered tools will increasingly assist clinicians in interpreting complex data from imaging, pathology, and genomics, enabling faster and more accurate diagnoses. For example, deep learning models are already rivaling radiologists in detecting early signs of diseases such as cancer. In primary care, AI chatbots and virtual assistants will help triage patients, monitor chronic conditions, and offer preliminary medical advice, reducing the burden on healthcare systems and allowing physicians to focus on more critical cases.

In surgery, AI will play a growing role in preoperative planning, intraoperative guidance, and postoperative care. Robotic surgical systems, enhanced by real-time AI analytics, will improve precision and minimize risks during procedures. Machine learning algorithms will assist surgeons by analyzing patient-specific data to predict complications and recommend optimal surgical strategies. Additionally, AI will streamline surgical workflows, automate routine documentation, and enable remote training through augmented reality and simulation platforms. These advances will not only increase surgical efficiency and safety but also help address workforce shortages and disparities in global surgical care.

The concern is 'garbage in' and garbage out. The data is only as good as how it is interpreted and what it actually means? Despite its limitless possibilities, the integration of AI into medicine over the next decade does not come without risks and challenges. One major concern is the potential for algorithmic bias, where AI systems trained on non-representative or flawed data may produce inaccurate or inequitable outcomes which could be more prevalent in rare diseases with limited data and also underrepresented populations. Healthcare professionals, once at the top of their game for skill, accuracy, knowledge and proficiency, may begin to lose their skillset and reduce their ability to make independent judgments in critical situations. Furthermore, issues around data privacy, security breaches, and the misuse of sensitive medical information could undermine patient trust. Inaccurate predictions or misdiagnoses by AI systems—especially if used without proper oversight—may result in harmful treatment decisions. Lastly, legal and ethical frameworks may struggle to keep pace with rapid technological advancements, leaving ambiguity around liability and accountability when AI-driven errors occur. AI must be handled with care; the human components of curiosity, a willingness to learn -creativity and logic can never be snuffed.

We are a more open-minded society as a whole, yet despite this information revolution, the healthcare industry has lagged behind with a "one-size-fits-all" approach to treating patients. ◦——➤ What vital truth are we missing when care is incomplete, nourishment is poor, and choices are limited? It's time we open our minds even more when it comes to taking charge of our own health, instead of placing undeserving trust in the very hands of those who are finding their way deeper and deeper into our pockets. Prescription medication is being used in larger numbers to treat various symptoms that are even more complex than that of patients past: obesity, anxiety, mental health, and post-traumatic stress disorder, to name a few. While allopathic medicine has its place in mainstream healthcare, overall, the industry approach has not evolved with the changing times of society. In fact, now pharmaceuticals are being joined with AI initiatives that may yield better diagnoses and enhanced monitoring, rather than getting to the root cause.

I recall a woman who came to the emergency department in obvious pain and discomfort, and upon examination, I noted she had severe end-stage breast cancer. Death was certainly imminent. Her chest was eaten away by ulcerous, oozing and decaying illness. I said to her, "why didn't you seek help sooner?" Her response was shocking: "I tried, but could not afford it!" She was admitted to the hospital that day, and for whatever reason, I felt the need to spend a few hours with her as she had nobody to turn to. I left the room well after midnight, and when I returned to the hospital the next day, she had died. Why does our current system allow this cruelty to occur to those in need? How is it that patients can accrue massive debts resulting in no other option than to declare bankruptcy due to unmanageable healthcare expenses? In fact, financial hardship due to healthcare debt is one of the leading causes of bankruptcy in the United States.

More than ever, symptoms observed in patient populations are becoming more diverse, thus creating a greater need for balance regarding treatment. In treating the patient, the provider may "win" or "lose," in treating an individual with customized, integrated solutions, the provider wins most of the time. Yet the current system essentially corners people into the "one-size-fits-all" space. It's not working, and it's not fair to everybody involved, mainly us consumers who are seeking better solutions.

You may notice the increase in chain pharmacies in your area, and they are popping up at an alarming rate. This is no coincidence as Big Pharma's voice and money is being put to use not only to line their pockets, but also to dictate the way in which healthcare is presented and perceived, with little or no regard to actual solutions to our health. The healthcare industry continues the trend of writing prescriptions for drugs and filling them without providing holistic/complementary options. There is an important piece of the puzzle missing when it comes to addressing the root causes. The current "band aid" approach places us at risk, while inherently procuring repeat customers through confusing and questionable tactics that not only promote dependency but also fail to address people's health as a whole. Other factors exist which could be mitigated through complementary care and not just allopathic care singularly, which get at the heart of the healthcare issue and fix it without draining finances and causing further deterioration in health.

There is an unprecedented amount of information available to us, and we certainly are a more abundant society, but are we healthier? Or at least, are we able to become healthier without breaking the bank? While there is more individual access to fresh water and food supplies in most regions, availability usually isn't the problem when it comes to products for sale at grocery stores. Rather, affordability is a key issue for those who are incapable of paying high prices for organic produce and for transportation to locations where there are fresh food options. It's interesting to note that a fast-food location may land on a street corner followed by its competition on the opposing corner, but, where's the fresh food market? A drive or a bus ride away!

Additionally, our quality of life could be exponentially enhanced with a more balanced offering, which should include knowledge and education at all levels. In many cases, it's simply a matter of not knowing. We've often asked people and colleagues why they are not eating healthy at lunch time and we hear it all: "I'm too busy", "All my friends go here", "It's cheaper", "I don't have time". Yet, to make and pack a gourmet sandwich or a fresh salad for lunch doesn't have to cost a lot and actually saves time when implemented.

It doesn't stop there, as voids still exist in healthcare equality, caused by multiple obstacles including, but not limited to, access to good jobs, schools, and safe, affordable homes. Health inequality should not be a topic in the day and age in which we live, but it remains a serious problem. According to the C.D.C., 6 of 10 adults have a chronic illness (Carney, 2023), approximately three-quarters of Americans are obese, and overweight, while mental illness and cancer in our youth is rising. C.D.C. data further suggests that 1 in 3 American teens are taking prescription medications, while at least 70 doses (and some reports indicate 90+) of 18 different vaccines from infancy until age 18 are recommended.

Why does the F.D.A. allow chemicals in U.S. foods and skincare products that are banned and outlawed in other countries? Depending on which studies you look at, approximately 200,000 patients die annually, and 400,000 hospitalized patients experience some difficulty and harm each year due to preventable medical treatment and medication errors. We'll save the discussion on the criminal-handling of the COVID 19 debacle for another day as more truths are still being revealed such as the number of sudden deaths occurring within 24-48 hours (as reported in VAERS) following a vaccination, Long Covid, and unseen research and data! Ideally, a system which offers more option-based alternatives would be a game changer in the lives of those who need it most, but this integrative path is being ignored, mainly because it would cut into the profits of those who are profiting most.

In the U.S., health insurance companies wield influence that reaches far beyond covering medical costs, effectively steering how care is delivered, priced, and accessed. Through reimbursement policies, coverage rules, and growing administrative requirements, insurers increasingly shape clinical decisions and financial viability across the system—trends that recent scrutiny of prior authorization practices and industry consolidation suggest may be undermining both patient care and provider stability.

The vicious cycle that is perpetuating a lot of this includes the money behind chemical medications. The harsh reality is that prescription drugs are good for the bottom line of Big Pharma companies. It's hard not to notice the increase in drug commercials on television that market so-called "cures" and "solutions" for ailments to the masses. You might also notice the double messaging throughout each commercial, which very quickly ticks off the possible side effects, while also portraying fun-filled, singing, dancing, and happy individuals. By themselves, the side effects should give us pause for thought. Some can be more ominous than the original symptom or ailment that the medication was prescribed to treat. Then there are the commercials that offer legal assistance in class action lawsuits against some of these very companies that marketed these drugs, knowing that there are patients who have not had relief from their pre-existing condition and now have some other ailment in which the alleged legal matter appears to match as the culprit. Yet most patients, greater than the age of 50 are taking at least 3-5 prescription medications. Additionally, despite decades of knowledge and evidence, chronic diseases and acute illness are often preventable with a natural diet of fresh foods, free from chemicals. Most medical schools still don't require a course in nutrition, and if they do, it's short in comparison to the barrage of pharmaceutical classwork and study being pushed, making holistic alternatives appear unimportant or even deemed irrelevant.

Technology and science are growing at exponential rates, resulting in new medical devices and mRNA-based pharmaceuticals which have changed how healthcare providers practice medicine, and even more disheartening, changing our views on what makes us sick, well, or healthy. Imagine for a moment that with all these brilliant advances in the medical field, perhaps the problem doesn't lie with technology or progress, but rather the lack of understanding about the nature of chronic illnesses. It's all very confusing and disheartening to consumers who are placing their trust in the healthcare system, while pharma is quick to discover new pathways for treatment where downstream effects are often unknown.

Moreover, the reported cost of medical errors and hospital-acquired infections is wide-ranging; it has been estimated to top the $20 billion+ mark annually. Depending on which reference you read, medical errors are between the first and third leading cause of death, while more than 70% of these are preventable (Croskerry, 2010). Millions of dollars are pumped into sophisticated research, yet the bar has not moved much in the way of progress, making us wonder if we are asking the right questions or are captured in an antiquated medical model that has yet to find itself. In the next chapter, we will explore steps we can take to reduce our risks of preventable diseases and illnesses and become proactive in our health outcomes, thus reducing potential medical errors and our dependence on high-cost medical treatments and prescription drugs.

CHAPTER 2:

"WHO SETS THE PRICE, WHO PAYS THE PRICE?"

As consumers and a society, we have been made to feel that we are powerless to fight the high cost of modern-day healthcare. Besides the potential cost to one's own health, there are inherent financial factors that drive up costs. The drug industry has become such a powerful entity that they can essentially call the shots when it comes to pricing! It is becoming difficult for the average household to keep up with the rising costs, especially if they have become dependent on certain medications that their insurance does not cover, or only covers a few brands, forcing the use of undependable or less studied generic formulations which are not mandated to stand up to the same rigors as name brands. If we were to estimate the number of new cancer cases in the USA per year to be approximately 2 million, that would mean that patients and families would be paying about $6 billion annually in out-of-pocket expenses, which further translates to $100-$200 thousand per patient for items such as surgery, radiation therapy, chemotherapy and other treatments. A HEALTH AND FINANCIAL CRISIS EXISTS NOW!! Insurance companies profit while patients go bankrupt!! Yet, the public in general is not recognizing the crisis exists, as the status quo has been slowly and strategically fed to us as "the only way," and it is cutting deeper than just the surface of socio-economic levels. Let's take it even one step further and emphasize that almost 90 percent of facilities manufacturing active pharmaceutical ingredients for medications intended for domestic US consumption are located outside the USA. So, what happens during challenging times – will Americans receive medications? This has been happening for some time now. As an example, quality issues with heparin and shortages of epinephrine have occurred throughout the years, but little has been done. America is now dependent on foreign nations to produce these key ingredients while losing independence and autonomy. Does this sound like America? And why, to save money while jeopardizing quality? This is a national security concern as domestic drug supply chains have to be protected from worldwide political disagreements, wars, tariffs, natural disasters, and cyberattacks.

Those who served in the military are experiencing the fallout of our current system, as well. For example, a veteran who fought for this country and now is home from deployment and suffering from PTSD may find it difficult to make a fair wage, much less receive adequate care within a VA system that once stood as a pillar of dependability and effectiveness. As a nation, we're dealing with an overburdened VA system (Kerfoot, 2024), which is negatively affecting the very people who put their lives at risk for the freedom and safety of the U.S. Essentially, as civilians, their lives are at risk once again. In many cases, these veterans have fallen victim to a VA system that is not only confusing to them, but due to a decrease in staffing, wait times to see doctors have lengthened, while facilities are not prioritizing them.

On a positive note, more veterans are enrolling into the VA health care system since the PACT Act of 2022, but the VA is now estimating that lack of funds for fiscal year 2025 approaches $7 billion. Imagine a veteran with post-traumatic distress disorder who desperately needs treatment in the way of medication and therapy but is not receiving the proper care and attention because their needs may not be addressed by a system with financial issues on top of everything else.. Remember, PTSD is not easy to treat, and medication alone does not solve the problem.

Completing forms and questionnaires is hard enough for a healthy individual let alone one who has been injured or experiencing mental illness. Although the VA has made strides in the way of updating their technology, many of the needs of veterans have been lost in the shuffle during this transition, while changes are ill-communicated and prove to be confusing. Vets continue to experience limited access to specialty care, and inadequate mental health staffing. There are misconceptions in how disability is determined based on specific questionnaires that need to be documented thoroughly and accurately, while requests may not only be denied due to minor errors and misinterpretations, but also resulting in unnecessary charges to our soldiers. Due diligence is still lacking to ensure cases are properly captured and documented. It's truly unimaginable when you think of the health effects that the anxiety alone brings to those who placed their lives on the line while answering the call of duty for our country, only to have added stress within a very confusing and inefficient process. Honorable lives are being lost unnecessarily, while those who should be prioritized are becoming irresponsibly forgotten.

Ethics and equality certainly come into the discussion, as the gap between the "haves and the have nots" is widening, putting further distance between who can and cannot afford to keep up with the cost of the very medication needed, or perceived to be needed. There is a disparity in the sharing of knowledge, as well, which could also impact people of all walks of life; the awareness of better options doesn't always reach those who need it most. Again, the "one-size-fits-all" approach does not take genetics, cultural diversities, and socio-economic factors into consideration. The current healthcare system doesn't work because it does not always address patients or their ailments on a case-by-case basis. It also fails to fulfill the person as a whole, which includes their mind, body, and spirit. What is good for one does not always guarantee it is good for another. "Recipe Book" medicine does not work! It's far more complex than that, but the solution doesn't come in one fell swoop. The answers must include a diverse spectrum of options in order to serve patients best, while presenting them in a way that can be easily understood, accessed, and afforded.

There is a level of individual responsibility when it comes to finding other ways to create a healthy balance to our lives and that of our family. At the very least, we should keep an open mind that there has to be a better way. However, it can be a daunting task with so much information and misinformation out there. It can also be discouraging financially on an individual basis, costs are simply outgrowing people's budgets. After all, why can't a family buy fruit and vegetables at a lesser cost than a meal from a fast food chain?! When did burgers and fries become the mainstream affordable food, and why are fast food places on every street corner, while families have to travel miles for fresh, organic food? There are reasons for this, too. Americans are paying more for healthcare than ever before, while this trend continues to rise at eye-opening rates. Our country spends more than $4 trillion a year on healthcare (Amin et al., 2025), which accounts for nearly 20% of the gross domestic product-- all while surprisingly lagging in the life expectancy category, compared to dozens of other countries. How does a "super power" nation such as ours consistently outspend just about every other nation per capita in the area of healthcare, while our life expectancy doesn't come close to reflecting this? The old system no longer works with a significantly growing population and massive immigration further challenging an already disconnected and broken healthcare landscape.

We, the consumers, are being dually attacked in the way of prescription drugs while questionable marketing campaigns push medication that hasn't been fully proven, may lack long-term data, and may not be necessary, or even safe. In many cases, medications are even being approved for children without sufficient data or testing. Pediatric patients have a unique vulnerability to adverse drug reactions, requiring caution during administration and monitoring to ensure safety and efficacy. Ask for more information and challenge instances where there may be potentially inappropriate use in all or a subgroup of pediatric patients.

While our food products are also cause for concern, not only do we have to be super diligent in what we choose to ingest medicinally, but even the meat we eat, vegetables we consume, and water we drink must be carefully chosen with an air of extreme caution. Animals are being injected with hormones and chemicals that find their way onto our dinner tables, while crops are being sprayed with pesticides and additives that are directly affecting our health and quality of life. Is that apple that we eat today, the same one that our grandparents ate? What has been lost in the way of nutrients, flavor, and nature? Since when did genetic and geo-engineering ever become part of a conversation or even the concept of edible vaccines which can be created by introducing a gene into a plant to manufacture an encoded protein? Possibly an even more important question is "what has been added to make 'it' unhealthy and unnatural?" Why would our government allow us to consume products that are largely affecting our health in negative ways? Like every great investigation or dive into finding answers there is the saying, "Follow the Money!"

We have come to believe that everything we see and hear about products we buy in the store has gone through a rigorous system of selection, with the stamp of approval from the FDA and others who are supposed to put our best interests at heart. But once again, the all-powerful dollar is the real inspiration behind what is put out there for our consumption. You may remember the popular snack campaign that included a slogan suggesting that you can't stop at just one? There is a reason why that goes beyond taste and satisfaction; and it lies in the fact that our so-called "snacks" and "treats" may be sprayed with chemicals not only to preserve their shelf lives, but with unnatural products to cause an addictive reaction amongst consumers (Bansal, 2022). Imagine the painstaking choice to spray both sides of each chip to promote more unhealthy consumption, which in turn provides more profit for the company. It's worth the company's time and effort to do this because it guarantees repeat customers for life. But at what cost to our health?

It's one thing to be a "label reader" when it comes to choosing products at the local grocery store, but it's altogether a different animal when warnings aren't provided for us in the way of the food chain. For example, does the meat we eat come with a disclaimer that the animal may have been raised unethically in inhumane conditions, while being impregnated with hormones that unhealthily increase their size in order to increase profits? Or does that apple we buy loosely at the store bother to include the chemicals that were sprayed on it in order to provide a more presentable color, while preserving its shelf life? What exactly are we putting into our bodies that is purposely being hidden from us? These questions must be asked before we take that next bite or swallow that next drink. If you cannot pronounce an ingredient that is unnatural…don't buy it!

This is not only a national crisis, but a familial and generationally traumatic issue that, if not challenged and changed, will affect not only our children, but our children's children, and so on. Our lives and quality of lives are at stake now, and we must regain control of our health and future. Childhood obesity is on the rise, childhood cancer is up, anxiety in young people is rising, one-third of teens in our country are ingesting prescription drugs (Tin, 2024), and almost 30% are pre-diabetic (Cooney, 2025). A staggering 18% of adolescents have nonalcoholic fatty liver disease. Yet we know that exercise invigorates and strengthens the heart, promotes circulation and brain health, reduces weight and cholesterol, and aids in preventing diabetes and heart disease. We as a country are failing our children with regard to healthcare, and a new norm is being established, while the status quo has been conditioned through commercials, government regulations, Big Pharma, and lack of knowledge of available and affordable alternatives.

Knowledge definitely is power, and ultimately we must empower ourselves in order to enact change. How does change happen when the odds are seemingly stacked against us? Well, one way is to change the landscape of the playing field; even though our nation has a broken healthcare system, we can individually shift our thoughts and actions to do our part within our own families. Well, what if we told you that you've already begun the process? "How?" you ask. The fact that you picked up this book for a reason should help answer your own question. In fact, your reasons for reading this are very closely linked with our reasons for writing it, and it lies in the shared belief that there must be a hopeful alternative—a better way! What if there already is a better way to choose your own integrative healthcare path that combines both holistic and allopathic choices, provides balance and vitality, and lowers your healthcare costs? We urge you to keep reading, keep asking questions, and keep on track as we walk this path together. We have already rolled up our sleeves and not only have we done extensive research for you, but we have spent the greater part of our adult lives developing that better way, with our CareXchange collective. The choice to become healthier just became easier, and less expensive.

Hint: "What would it mean to reclaim ownership of your health decisions?

CHAPTER 3:

"FOOD FOR THOUGHT"

In coming years, total health care expenses are expected to account for 25% of the U.S. Gross Domestic Product (GDP), and even with the Affordable Care Act (ACA), more than 27 million Americans still lack health insurance (Insurance Newsnet, 2024). More than half of Americans (51%) now have trouble handling out-of-pocket insurance expenses (Commonwealth Foundation 2023), according to a survey by the Commonwealth Foundation. Therefore, total health care costs must be addressed head on, rather than kicking the can down the road and passing the buck and cost burdens to insurers, hospitals, providers, patients or even government, as it will not solve the problem of unsustainable healthcare costs.

We are entering into a new age of transformation and healthcare revolution because Americans are realizing the manipulation of the system with minimal improvement in health. How many real life examples are required that depict patients going to see their providers, or having to go to the hospital for surgery, only to be placed on multiple medications with no improvement post-surgery while many times experiencing even worse effects than when they first reached out for help? An uprising is occurring in the realization of alternative therapies that go beyond a failed system—taking charge of our health and the drive for better results. We will describe alternative therapies in a later chapter as it goes well beyond taking a multi-vitamin and thinking that will suffice! After all, what does taking that vitamin actually do for you outside of checking the "oh, I'm healthy now" box? How do you even know these supplements are right for you?

It has been said that, "People don't care how much you know until they know how much you care." This mantra has been our driving force, as we've prided ourselves on living both our professional and personal lives in a manner which serves others best. Caring is at the very core behind the countless hours of studying, research, and continuous education that we've done, and will continue to do, as we fervently pursue answers that will have a positive impact on as many people as possible. We are "walking the walk" together!

I grew up around my aunts and uncles who smoked, worked in coal mines, and survived the depression years. I watched my relatives "graduate" secondary to cancer and heart disease. My father passed after having multiple strokes. This gave me the fortitude to push forward into healthcare so I could, in turn, make a difference. While witnessing the experiences of many patients with trauma, and acute and chronic illness, I have noted some who made it through their health challenges, when all the facts pointed to a certain demise. This phenomenon begs the question, "Why?" What was the dimension and realm that made this occur? We'll get into that later, too! So, after all the schooling and exposure to patient care, it became clear that the current system certainly wasn't cutting it. May I remind you that 30 million Americans are without health insurance, which, in turn, limits their access to affordable, high-quality care? Therefore before we go too deep, this chapter is about the solution and the revolution.

Picasso may have been the one who said, "Find your gift, then give it away." Well, we have found our gift in this life, both in clinical experience, as well as in the educational realm, and we believe it is our purpose and obligation to share what we've learned with others, in hopes that it will enhance their/your life as much as it has ours. Yes, purpose and passion are our catalysts, and it is our sincere hope that it sparks something inside you to cultivate a mindset and approach to life that is characterized by awareness, presence, faith and well-being.

In order to break down the walls of change and shift the paradigm, there must be an open mind, followed by a burning desire, through a belief system that will not stop seeking a better way of doing things, regardless of the obstacles. Just think for a moment of when we were born, not knowing, not being exposed to toxins ex-utero, in essence—perfect. Then we crawl, eat baby food, and breastfeed, or drink milk (or imitation). We eventually learn to walk, while experiencing scrapes, cuts, and bruises from falling down. Possibly even more, in the way of broken bones, injuries, automobile accidents, emotional issues—okay, I'll stop there for now. The bottom line is how did we go from a beautiful healthy baby, perfect in every way, to having disease? Is it possible that we are indeed the paradoxical shift—our minds, bodies, and spirits, coupled with the divinity to which we are surrounded are in constant motion?

If our body responds to our environment, our thoughts, our food, our drink—then our health can be transformed! According to Earl Nightingale, "We become what we think about," and we must make a conscious decision to enact change. We will go deeper into this in later chapters, but is it possible that by being created in the image of God, we already possess the ability to aid in our own treatments and health journey? In S. I. McMillen's book entitled None of These Diseases (McMillen, S.I., & Stern, D. 2000), McMillen describes a biblical footprint on how to optimize our health by following the laws of scripture and what the Bible advises us to eat. What if we went beyond just our physical self with the realization that quantum physics is real? The molecular-biology model is based on old principles which are proven by fact that some patients survive a specific illness, yet others do not, even though treatments and disease states were the same. Certainly, there is more.

Current care networks still fail to take into consideration emotional states, the power of mindful consciousness, and the energy and life force of our very spirit and soul. There are multi-dimensional aspects to health that turn bodily functions, cells, receptors, and feedback loops on and off outside of pharmaceutics. For example, clinical hypnosis has gained growing recognition as a scientifically supported, non-drug intervention grounded in established neurobiological mechanisms. It represents a low-cost, low-risk approach that has demonstrated therapeutic benefit without reliance on specialized technology, and it shows adaptability across diverse patient populations and clinical environments. "What? How is this possible?" you may wonder. This idea is referred to by some as vibrational medicine and bioenergetics, but it goes much farther and deeper beyond this. Even the concepts behind electro-magnetic healing evoke questions that remain unanswered by modern medicine. Medical philosophy can't even address the simple questions of what is life and who am I? How can a salamander regenerate a limb but not a human? We haven't even touched the surface! Empowerment is our responsibility while we seek knowledge and solutions. Yes, knowledge is definitely power, and when backed by action and belief, it becomes a super power!

While on our quest to disrupt the current healthcare system, with all its inherent inequities, we have been driven to seek and identify solutions for those who are seeking to take control of healthcare costs in the most affordable way possible, through a cost-sharing community. With access to this community, people from all walks of life feel encouraged and have a sense of belonging, while empowered to choose the very best options when it comes to their health. Through a simple, yet diversified, integrative approach based on personal needs, preferences, genetics, and background, a community-driven system fulfills the needs of individuals and families, all while controlling costs. This synergistic approach lessens the overall out-of-pocket expense, while the burden of cost is shared and spread out amongst many, instead of one.

Given the dividedness of our political system and the huge financial debt of our nation, it will be sometime down the road before serious and comprehensive healthcare insurance reform is put in motion. Rather, it is likely that more emphasis will be placed on individual states to drive consumer awareness, and aid in driving costs down. It has become quite clear that the current healthcare finance and quality is the real problem, and it's getting worse! High administrative costs, uncontrolled chronic conditions, increasing mental health issues, and a blatant disregard for preventing life-threatening conditions, set the tone. To achieve a high performing, value-based, quality health system, perplexing problems such as access, quality, and cost must be overcome, while institutions must also come together as "one!" This is how things got done years ago—driving political and economic change with one voice!

Imagine a community--and for the sake of visuals—a setting back in time in an open farm-like area whereby neighbors come together to build a house for a family. First, there is someone who knows engineering and draws out a plan and does the measurements while others gather necessary materials. Then a woodworker provides the wood and ability to cut the proper angles and fittings. A plumber designs the proper piping and irrigation system. There are plenty of helping hands for the lifting and nailing, while others run back and forth for supplies, and food to feed the workers. Add some landscapers who create an agreeable outside appearance with regard to foliage, grass, and walkway. The garden is then put in place, while seeds are planted for future harvests. Others grab some paint and begin painting a fence that they just installed, while some paint the outside framework. Now it's coming together, and as days go by, dressing up the inside with modest decorations and furniture is next. Before long, raw materials have been transformed into a house, and now it has become a home all because integrative building blocks came together through a pooling of resources from many. The sharing of this, as well as the workload, has made it feasible.

"It takes a village" in creating something wonderful, whether raising a child, building a home, and even bettering one's physical and financial health. There is something very beautiful and unique that happens when we share. We created CareXchange because we wanted to help. We wrote this book because we felt not only a need to bring awareness to those who need it, but also because our lives and your lives are worth it. Together, we can remind each other of the importance of God's love, balance, nutrition, self care, vitality, and a positive outlook as we live our best lives possible.

Now take the same building block example of creating a home from raw materials and community effort and imagine picking and choosing components to create the best formula possible for your well-being, including but not limited to nutrition. Now add holistic enhancements to alleviate stress, like yoga or meditation, to help lower blood pressure, and exercise to enhance vascular tone. We can draw from the best of both worlds, too, with Western medicine merging with Eastern practices, while achieving the maximum result.

Historically, patients' challenges have stemmed from either lack of knowledge and/or lack of options, as allopathic practices usually only offer one choice, in the way of medication. In the words of Will Rogers, "the problem in America isn't so much what people don't know; the problem is what people think they know that just ain't so." There are natural options for most of the ailments facing society, and when there are not, at least a combined effort of a complementary strategy to address root causes can not only be more effective, but more cost-effective. When it comes to the health and prosperity of you and your families, the shift of power will now return to where it belongs...back in your hands!

More than ever before, it is imperative that we contribute wholeheartedly to our body, mind, and spirit, while we face not only challenges within the healthcare system, but also navigate through unprecedented health conditions. It is not only our responsibility; it is the greatest gift to ourselves to nurture our whole self, through knowledge, nutrition, and self-care. Our proactivity and our voice are pillars to the very foundation of our longevity and quality of life, as we remind ourselves, and each other, that our body truly is a very special and unique temple--a beautiful gift from God!

Back to the example of the house—can we agree that having a community that fosters wellness and works together is stronger? Imagine a patient who does not know about a condition, who blindly goes to their medical provider, versus the patient who is part of a community network that is informed and able to navigate the health scenario. This is real. There is a lack of understanding, documentation, communication, and guidance throughout the patient experience. After all, who is protecting the rights, quality care, and education of the patient? Remember the Hippocratic Oath, "Do no harm?" There needs to be a patient-centered approach which empowers through knowledge, strengthens by action, and sustains through community. We're also experiencing an I.T. revolution with new technologies arriving each day and living in an ever-changing world. An important step will be how data is incorporated and strategically implemented to drive better outcomes and save costs. During the Covid pandemic, telemedicine use in clinical care became extremely accessible while demonstrating huge value.

The community needs to be aligned with the notation that our overall health goes beyond face value, as well as beyond the current health presentation of using only pharmaceuticals which may only be masking the very symptoms to which root causes need to be identified, or else illness may continue to progress without resolution. Congratulations on achieving Level 1!! In the next chapter, we will explain CareXchange and why it is important to start getting into healthier patterns and solutions.

Hint: If nutrition is foundational to health, is what you eat contributing to your healing or harm?

NOW ENTERING LEVEL 2:

Power & Choice

CHAPTER 4:

"SEEKING SOLUTIONS"

It has become increasingly obvious that the life-changing process of choosing what's in our best interest regarding a health regimen needs to be determined by those who will be most greatly affected by such a crucial decision: ourselves! The current healthcare climate is continually and strategically shifting from a patient-first, case- by-case, root-cause plan of action, when it comes to treatment options-- to a monopolistic, ulterior-motived, and even dangerously controlled landscape, by those who have made it abundantly clear that our best interests are not being placed first.

Dorothy and I were speaking with a neighbor recently who described the ongoing seizure disorder of a loved one, and, it was not until recently, when a doctor from EU was visiting and asked to see the patient. He quickly realized that while the patient had been exposed to every anti-seizure medication known to man, that nobody had bothered to check ammonia levels. When the lab work came back, the ammonia levels were astonishingly high and when treated, with simple low-cost solutions, the seizure activity minimized. Until recently, our options were limited by health insurance usually provided through our employer, or if self-employed, at an even larger out-of-pocket expense. Employer- sponsored insurance made available through an "open season" enrollment period offers health coverage to employees without "specific-to-our-need choices." Limited by its own devices, employers usually pay a percentage of the coverage, while the employees are responsible for the rest, which is usually the bulk of the cost. We've been programmed to believe not only is this the only way, but through a conditioning of acceptance, there is an air of subservient gratitude that such an offering is made available to us in the first place, as it is considered a benefit for employment. We have all had conversations with people who state the only reason their loved one is working is for health insurance. Is that a ball and chain? And if so, where is the quality of life, and, if there is limited quality of life will health be jeopardized? Typically, our bi-weekly payroll check would be dinged for a percentage of the cost to carry medical insurance. For some, this is an "out-of-sight, out-of-mind" scenario as the true cost becomes fogged up and lost in the shuffle within the confusing fine print details of the insurance itself and if the paycheck is high enough, little attention is focused on insurance costs. How about the reverse—an employee making under $50,000 annually may see the amount being taken for insurance as hypocrisy, unfair, abusive and cruel?

Once the coverage is active, and an employee makes an appointment to see their medical provider, a co-payment out-of-pocket cost is paid for the services of seeing the provider. Depending on the specific situation, diagnosis, etc., a prescription is written to alleviate the symptoms of the patient. Then a visit to the pharmacy is next, and possibly another out of pocket cost for the remaining balance of the medication that is not covered through insurance. Most of us are very familiar with these processes as employees, or former employees, within a traditional healthcare system. It's also an example of an allopathic approach to healthcare, whereby a diagnosis is made, based on symptoms, followed by an order/prescription for chemical medication for the patient to take to mitigate the symptoms.

Some of the inherent challenges that we face as a nation when it comes to traditional healthcare insurance include inadequate coverage, cost concerns, lack of specialty care, and the complexity and confusion of how it all works. Furthermore, inadequacies within the system leave some people exposed to future medical debt. Not all plans are created equally, and for those who find this out too late, it could mean both under coverage, which will weigh heavily on their pockets, peace of mind, as well as an overall emotional and financial insecurity, which in turn, may add to health woes. Hence: the makings of a vicious cycle begins.

Like we mentioned in an earlier chapter, our veterans are facing challenges when it comes to specialty care, and this is not exclusive to our flawed VA system, as it's a serious concern throughout the employer-based coverage for many civilians, as well. Those who are suffering mental health challenges like anxiety, PTSD, depression, and other nuanced healthcare needs could be exposed to the harsh reality of being underinsured through the traditional plans which require extra out-of-pocket costs.

Other financial concerns can be found within the shocking statistic that half of insured adults are stressed about being able to afford their health insurance monthly premiums and even consider their coverage as "fair" or "poor" due to high out-of-pocket costs for doctor visits. These concerns inherently affect our overall health and quality of life as we've been boxed in far too long!

Even more staggering is that a paltry nine percent of people understand the terms of premium, deductible, co-insurance, and out-of-pocket maximum. The vast majority of employees/participants don't understand the very health insurance that they pay for and rely on for their well-being. Herein lies the problem with traditional health insurance: they're simply too complicated and/or designed in such a manner that participants are confused to the point where they are paying for services that are not fully realized—thus, keeping the costs down for the employers/providers but not the patient. Because of the confusion, planned designs within such coverage that may potentially offer some financial incentives, are baffling consumers to the point where they aren't sure what the true costs are, so they can't maximize any savings. Whether the vague, complex, and confusing nature of these models are purposely written that way or not, it's nonetheless disconcerting to the consumer who is left with the short end of the stick.

This frustration can evolve into fear from uncertainty, which leads people to remain stagnant and not seek treatment when needed. For example, 44 percent of Americans have avoided getting healthcare services because they were unsure of the costs (HealthSparq, 2022). Progression of such diseases as diabetes and heart disease can become more serious when untreated which in turn, diminishes the overall quality of life, and can potentially lead to death. There is an overall dissatisfaction among plan members, and those who need it most are at the greatest risk. When we take into consideration peace of mind, quality of life, and the overall health risks involved within the traditional ways of healthcare, what are the true costs we are incurring? How can we give ourselves a better chance of overall health within a system that has consistently reared weaknesses within its very foundation, while increasing costs that are breaking our banks?

Now we are seeing grassroots efforts, along with a growing number of physicians and specialists who have realized this inadequacy, and are moving away from traditional healthcare insurance reimbursement models in favor of more transparent, affordable, cash-based services. Frustrated by rising administrative costs, limited patient interaction time, and opaque pricing tied to insurance companies, these providers are embracing direct-pay or membership-based models that offer patients lower costs and clearer value. This shift often includes simplified pricing structures, direct primary care (DPC), telemedicine, and specialized services offered at a fraction of insurance-billed rates. The movement aims to restore autonomy to providers while improving access, affordability, and trust for patients, particularly those with high-deductible plans or no insurance at all.

It's not about 'bucking' the system; rather, the realization that the system is not working and therefore exploring a different path cannot be denied. For example, a "teamwork makes the dream work" methodology. Cost sharing for healthcare is a cutting-edge way to offset costs as you pay less for a more diverse, nurturing, and specific-to-your-need approach, which is all within your control. While it is cutting edge, as explained earlier, this concept is not new but now much more refined. Within a very organized and easy to understand format, cost sharing through CareXchange unites patients, doctors, treatments, wellness and guidance options.

CareXchange is not health insurance, rather it is an option that aids in keeping healthcare costs under your own control, within your budget, and aligned more specifically to who you are as a whole person within your body, mind, and spirit. By its core definition, health cost sharing provides a collective approach to aid in paying for medical care. However, it's much more than that because of the broad array of additional options made available to each participant, including alternative, integrative, and holistic possibilities. This is what makes CareXchange unique.

Beyond a fiscally responsible model regarding healthcare, cost sharing is an open-minded approach to treatment within an ever-changing, complex, and challenging health landscape. The broad spectrum of illnesses facing our nation today requires a myriad of options that are as unique as the person/persons for which they're intended. Remember, if the "root cause" is addressed rather than the "Band-Aid" approach of chasing symptoms, the result will be a more satisfying and cost-effective approach to wellness, vitality and overall quality of life. While cost sharing offers an overall peace of mind financially, it also makes available to like and fair-minded participants a community-oriented alignment that shares information for the sake of educating and informing to avail optimal results. There's definitely a power-in-numbers approach that gives participants the ability, and access, to their health choices in an integrative manner. Integrative medicine pairs Western/conventional (traditional allopathic) medicine with other treatments (Alternative medicine) such as acupuncture, chiropractic, massage therapy, etc., to assuage symptoms, pain, and side effects.

Health challenges go far beyond the physical ailments that affect us; there are mental, emotional, and psychological variances we all face that impact our overall health. Mental health issues are rising in America as people are attempting to adapt to a world that is moving faster than ever, with dynamics never before seen, or addressed, and the evolution of healthcare must heed the call of our changing times. These challenges, too, need to be recognized within treatment options because one is just as important as the other when we are talking about our body, mind, and spirit (Holistic).

There has been a level of ignorance, apathy, and naivety when it comes to our conditioning and perceived dependence regarding a Western Medicine-only mentality. Some of this is not our fault as this has been generationally force-fed to us over time. Eastern Medicine cannot, and should not, be excluded when it comes to healthy alternatives, as it dates back over 3,000 years. The staying power of natural healing methods speaks volumes to Holistic Medicine's credibility, and when combined with the possibilities that Western Medicine technologies offer, it can provide extremely powerful solutions.

The early evidence of cost sharing in healthcare dates to the 1900's as close-knit communities would support each other financially during times of need. This is evidenced by Amish and Mennonite families in the United States pooling their money/resources together to help each other during trying times. Additionally, the process has been a slow but steady evolution over the last century as Christian cost-sharing ministries have continued to evolve. Again, with the changing times of our nation's health (and world, for that matter), it has become necessary to fine tune the cost-sharing concept in order to maximize its benefits to today's generation. ⚷ What small step today returns the power of health and well-being to your hands? Ultimately, our health is our responsibility, and the purpose of this book is to convey awareness.

Moreover, your financial, physical, emotional, psychological, and holistic well-being can be greatly enhanced as you will realize a better way of choosing your own healthcare solution that suits your specific needs, all while providing the peace of mind, and quality of life you so vitally deserve! Our next chapter will delve into something that already exists inside of you waiting to be discovered, uncovered, and awakened!

CHAPTER 5:

"EMPOWERMENT"

*"The two most important days in your life are the day you are born
and the day you find out why."*

--Mark Twain

Have you ever asked, "Why am I here?" Or "What is my purpose in life?" Or even, "What path do I choose?" Do you ever ask a child what they want to be when they grow up? Do you remember when you were asked the same question? Exploring our thoughts and intentions through information we are exposed to (as well as that which we are not), within our spiritual beings, empowers us to explore our options, and implement "optimal thinking." Our intentions can be quite powerful when they are realized. Many actors/actresses, musicians, vocalists, and sports figures did not get to where they are by letting the world go by—rather it was through manifestation, as well as a presence and awareness of their capabilities. Some may be born with natural talent, but left untapped and unchallenged, it will atrophy like a limp muscle. This realization comes from learning, open mindedness, and awareness. A mental change has to occur that inspires courage, commitment, focus, and desire. But where does this drive and passion come from?

More than a word, empowerment can be a movement, a testament, and an overall energy source. We've probably heard the word itself more in the last decade than ever before, as it has become somewhat of a tagline within the personal development realm. This is not to say its validity is any less interesting or important than the first time we may have heard it. In fact, if we take a moment to break down its true definition, only then can we derive the very essence of its strength and hopefully apply its concept to our own life. The more we understand its true meaning, the more we'll appreciate it and then coax our potential through it. The process of giving people the power to make decisions and act on their own behalf (Merriam-Webster, n.d.). Empowerment can refer to the level of autonomy and self-determination that people and communities have, but more importantly, what they do with autonomy. An applicable reference to what we've been discussing can be found in the previous chapter. Since it has become increasingly apparent that the motives behind government, Big Pharma, and the healthcare industry as a whole are not serving us in a manner that is protective, economical, or even very safe, it is more incumbent upon ourselves than ever before to be self-governing when it comes to our own well-being.

How exactly do we begin to empower ourselves, our health, and that of our families? You've already heard the phrase, "Knowledge is power" and you'll hear it throughout this book because knowledge and awareness are the cornerstone of self-empowerment. You'll be able to add the necessary weaponry of knowledge to your arsenal in order to navigate through the confusing and slippery slopes of the healthcare industry, while enacting change in yourself, thus enhancing your quality of life, and peace of mind. Through awareness and knowledge, we begin the process of understanding that will help piece together a belief system that provides the strength and momentum to accomplish that which we aspire.

Congratulations! You are gaining some essential awareness through the information in this book, which has been amassed through countless hours of passionate research and experience. The next step of your self-empowerment health journey is literally your first step. Like any great challenge, change, or adventure, it begins one step at a time.

One of the most important questions we can ask ourselves is, "What is our why?" We all have a "why:" that reason we work toward something, that driving force in our lives, some thing or things that are unequivocally the most important to each of us, why we do the things we do, what our inspiration/motivation is, and things that drive us to do more. For most people, their "why" may be the person or people whom they love. A mother/father who works hard and sets a positive example so that their children may experience stability and habits that will empower them to do the same for themselves and their future children as well, is certainly an honorable pursuit, and a great example of a "why". For some, it might be a passion project of giving their time, energy or money through philanthropy. Some may be motivated by finances, recognition, and/or lifestyle. We toiled, labored, strived and persevered in our pursuit to become a doctor and nurse because our "why" was, and still is, to help others heal and improve their quality of life. Our "why" continues to evolve as do we, so that we can provide information to our readers, family, and friends, as well as participants of the community.

Define your reason for making that change in you, and your life will become that change! Your answer to your own quest or question will be your purpose-driven mission and the continuous motivation to keep going. Entropy is a movement from order to disorder with the thought that as the surrounding becomes more disorganized, it is actually becoming organized. Otherwise stated, it is a measure of how many possible options exist that correspond to something you can actually see or visualize. Although entropy has been commonly used in thermodynamics, it can be applied to almost anything in theory: a model airplane that comes in pieces, a building block set, construction plans and more. Now, for those that do not clean our rooms but for some reason we know the location of one yellow sticky note within a stack of papers, this may sound entertaining, but let's take a moment to reflect on what we can't see. Energy exists all around us in different forms, and according to Newton's 1st Law of Thermodynamics, can neither be created nor destroyed. But we know it's there. How? Look at how the wind makes a tree branch move—that's a transfer of energy and mass. This became the basis of flight along with Bernoulli's principle which we won't go into here.

Quantum physics speaks to the small particles in motion that we cannot see, but we know exist. Just check out a drop of water or blood under a high-powered microscope. A red blood cell has a typical diameter between 6.2 to 8.2 micrometers! It would take 13 million red blood cells lined up one next to another to stretch across a 100 yard football field! We also know about even smaller protons, electrons, and atoms—all of which we cannot see, that, in addition to biomolecular pathways, allow cells to communicate with one another. What if there was an additional dimension added to this dynamic? Perhaps a spiritual dimension and life force, where once accessed, all cells and energy achieved balance? Imagine what that can do for health. We'll get into this even more in Chapter 13. Have you ever had an experience where everything just seemed to come together perfectly, and you said, "Well, that was pretty amazing?!" Whether running a race, baking a cake, giving a presentation, working on a house, or any undertaking, for that matter, a feeling of flooded energy from within the body and beyond propels you to another level.

Our health is being influenced by what we cannot see. The Bible mentions that we strive according to His energy that powers us. The triad of mind, body, and spirit creates a virtual, multi-dimensional force field that leads to empowerment and better health. This state of awareness is where everything becomes clear, and the path is revealed. Everything comes together and just makes sense. Remember, we become what we think about. In the movie "The Matrix," Keanu Reeves became aware of space and time and was able to move through it. His character moved from one door to the next allowing him to travel outside normal space, but some doors were locked, representing freedom versus resistance like gateways to deeper understanding, power, and responsibility (Wachowski & Wachowski, 1999). Our intentions are important, and if our beings exist beyond time and space, and interact with multiple forms of energy, then do we have the power to change our health status? Yes! As an example, let's take the individual who is harboring anger from a job or depression from a breakup, both of which may result in rapid heartbeat, restlessness, dyspepsia, nausea, diarrhea, back pain, and headaches. Fatigue sets in, along with depression while the anger continues. Increased heart rate drives hypertension and headaches lessen clarity of thought.

Next, because of lack of concentration, an exam was just flunked, a presentation in the office failed and the last check to the bank was missed. This is a downward spiral, and we all have experienced it in one way or another. This spiral, if left unchanged, can impact the rest of our lives. Now let's introduce empowerment and allow multiple dimensions of energy to create awareness and lessen anger and depression. What will likely happen to these symptoms? You got it! They will lessen, and may even disappear altogether. And what about the exam, the presentation and the check? All a success!

You may be saying, "It's too late for me, as I've treated my body horribly over the years. I smoke, drink, I have stress, I work in a crummy job, and won't change." In essence, this is health inequity, a culturally driven setting which is not limited to, but more commonly observed in low-income areas, those with mental illnesses, teens with peer pressure, and families where poor health is common. But, this is also seen in the rich and famous. As wealth is accumulated, there is also time to think and if the mind and body are unable to cope with the success and it is not filling a " purpose," a gaping hole is left—yearning for attention which so often becomes filled by the turmoil of addiction.

During my early medic years, I picked up the remains of a patient who shot himself in the head with a 12-gauge shotgun and left a suicide note which read, "Start an I.V. of Budweiser, and leave me to die!" Similarly, I cut down a young adolescent from a tree limb after hanging himself all because he got a "C" on an exam and he was scared, upset and did not want to face his family. Certainly, there must be a better way!

Another important note to your "why" is a follow up question of "why not?" Especially when talking about empowerment and possibilities, this question actually becomes a statement as we open our minds to find better options. "Some men see things as they are and say why, I dream things that never were and say why not." (Back to Methuselah, 1949, p. 7).This famous quote from a George Bernard Shaw play is a powerful reminder of imagining a better way, world, and life. The spirit of open-mindedness is empowering in itself because it flows continuously and is ever-evolving to not only find answers, but to put them to action. Instead of a closed mind that ceases to allow new information in, stunting any possible solution or growth. Open minds have always been the catalyst for the great innovators, inventors, scientists, and philosophers of our world. As we created CareXchange, we were driven by both the questions and statements within "why/why not?" We started with the root cause of why the health care industry was broken, mismanaged, badly intended, greedy and unfair, and we went to work with open minds of finding solutions through a "why not?" process.

Consider your quest for longevity and health prosperity to be your own personal journey, and most importantly, an adventure that will ultimately lead you to the promised land. That proverbial pot of gold at the end of the rainbow will be in the form of a life well-lived and fully realized for you and your family. Through asking questions, finding answers, and processing information that better serves your decision-making process, you can and will become the best version of yourself! Beyond reading labels on food items in the grocery stores, which in itself is paramount, find the best and most cost-effective ways to improve your health through nutrition. In previous chapters, we've discussed food, and what you may see at the chain grocery stores, so it's of utmost importance that you discover organic food options that have been grown without pesticides, preservatives, additives, hormones, and genetic manipulation. If you have land available, start small and plant a garden. If there is a back deck or patio available, there are portable and stackable garden options. Hippocrates is credited with stating, "Let thy food be thy medicine." Will this require work? The simple answer is yes! But you'll find that healthier alternatives are out there if you're willing to find them, and the benefits far outweigh the efforts and costs, both fiscally and physically.

It is amazing to realize that Hippocrates, who lived in approximately 460 B.C., realized that disease is not an entity, but a fluctuating condition of the body—a battle of sorts between the substance of the disease and the natural self-healing tendency of the body. Modern medicine in its shift to Big Pharma and medical devices still have not learned this invaluable lesson, and if they do, there is little effort to reinforce this aspect of wellness. We know how people die, but we still do not fully understand why people die. Self-healing is up to us, along with the awareness that empowers us to work harder to achieve better health. The decision is ours because this goes beyond where current medicine can take us.

Depending on your particular medical situation and/or diagnosis, research the root cause of what ails you. Oftentimes, there are alternatives to prescription drugs. Before you opt for chemical drugs through that next prescription, find out why it was prescribed in the first place and possibly attack it from a homeopathic stance. The same exists for surgery—depending on what news you hear on any day, unnecessary surgeries occur between 10-25% of the time costing the healthcare system 750 billion dollars annually. Again, the path to wellness is a step-by-step approach that is realistically doable and applicable with every little positive change going toward results and feeling better. If you're overweight, and begin a moderate walking regiment, you'd be pleasantly surprised at how quickly your endurance level improves, as well as the chain of goodness that comes to you in the form of lowering your blood pressure, mental health/ clarity, purpose, improved energy, and weight loss. If you were taking medications for some of the ailments tied into being overweight, shockingly enough those may be alleviated and even eliminated. We are now becoming aware of individuals taking a "skinny shot" who are not prepared to "see" themselves as skinny, leading to a whole mess of other issues.

Many of us may be aware of serotonin, which exists naturally in our body and acts as a neurotransmitter, and referred to as the "happy chemical." Serotonin and melatonin play a key role in regulating mood, sleep, appetite and other bodily functions. A simple change in exercise and nutrition can turn on serotonin like a light switch and improve other areas of your life. This is self-empowerment and self-improvement at its finest, and it didn't cost you anything but time, which is our greatest asset. Moreover, you didn't have a body part removed from surgery. When one vital organ is removed, it places more burden on remaining systems, and possible pharmaceutical/ chemical dependency for life with its absence. This is not undermining modern medicine and science as we also note that sometimes surgeries cannot be avoided, but, this should be a last resort and not a first choice without first considering all the options. Our bodies were designed by God. All bodily systems have a specific purpose and act in tandem with each other, making us the divine human beings we are. Most of us already know what we can do to make an impact on our health yet find unlimited excuses and reasons not to act.

Could it be fear? If so, what's the answer?: Face Everything And Recover because uncertainty is part of life. Once we empower ourselves with the right information that serves us best, we can implement this into action. We've also been greatly misled with the "quick fix" approach through big pharma as the best option and only way. We can and should be our greatest health advocate and advisor because it is a matter of life and death.

Read about Eastern Natural Medicinal alternatives too, and apply these forms of self-care to your life. Make sure to take into consideration what is right for you based on tolerances, allergies, age, etc., and see how you look and feel compared to your earlier self. Learn about meditation, yoga, breathwork, herbs, and more, while giving them a try. Invest in yourself through a once-in-awhile massage, facial, retreat, and you'll be glad you did. Go for a walk in a park, go to the zoo—do something different and shift your behavior. When we change our behavior our perspective also changes. There isn't only one way to make change, and it doesn't have to be painful

THE LIFE WELLNESS COLLECTIVE

or very costly. In fact, a morning stretch, a community class, a book, a soul-fulfilling experience often costs very little, or nothing at all. Self-care is not only an integral part of our physical health-- but it serves our soul, as well. Remember, we are on a quest to improve our whole selves including body, mind, and spirit. Our CareXchange philosophy allows for you to tap into the resources necessary that hit on all points, all while lowering your costs and honoring the living, breathing gift which is you!

We've been force-fed information with narratives that have ultimately served the dictates and profits of a monopolistic healthcare system for years now, while our health and quality of life remains at stake. There is no greater tool than the one we have in our possession, and that is the power to choose what is best for ourselves and create our own path, joined by a multi-dimensional, quantum matrix of energy, steered by the power of God.. Good people have fought and died for our freedom, some are family and very close friends (which I also call family). The battle cry and flame of freedom cannot be extinguished and makes this country great. The song of 'America' is clear: "My Country 'Tis' of Thee, sweet land of liberty, of thee I sing; Land where my fathers died, Land of the pilgrim's pride, From every mountainside Let freedom ring". Now, good people are dying unnecessarily, because somewhere along the way, our "health" vision has been strategically blurred by those who are placing greed over need, and profit over people, when it comes to healthcare in America. Let us not be fooled anymore, and let's take control of our life and health once and for all.

Do you know your "Why?" If not, that's okay but look for signs—listen to "God's Whisper" and it will appear. It can be heard in so many ways: the silent voice in our heads when we wake up in the morning, a phone call from a neighbor in need, a problem at work or at home, a promotion, graduation and more! A whisper can be subtle and it can also be mind-blowing! Something that triggers us to say, "I need to change" and "this is not right." After all, how is it that we are the only beings on earth that understand right and wrong? There are seven key steps to empowerment that also involve our rights to our freedom of health, speech, and religion. We have the right to choose our path. The first step is responsibility—your decision for better health starts with you! Nobody can do it for you. The second step involves setting realistic goals, and taking one day at a time. The third step is education—take time to learn and establish a game plan. The fourth step is taking action—no time like the present. The fifth step is monitoring your progress—check in and ask yourself, "How am I doing?" The sixth step is to realize the journey—it's not easy, but stay motivated, as it is okay to take two steps forward and one step back. The last key step is to forgive yourself—stay committed with the realization and awareness you've gained. Remember, knowledge equals empowerment, and taking that first step to regaining control of your body, mind, and spirit is one of the most powerful things you can do!

Now that we've established that due diligence equals "you diligence," and that the question "why?" can lead to the even more powerful question/statement "why not?" What are you going to do with this information? Let's take this ride together and continue the path of empowering ourselves as seekers of knowledge and truth.

Not by the information that we've been force-fed all these years, but the real, raw truth through case studies, as well as centuries of natural remedies as alternative therapies. Stay tuned!

🌿 Reflection Question: How is your empowerment connected to your wellness?

CHAPTER 6:

FREEDOM OF CHOICE

Before we give away the prize, let's get into health cost sharing. We talked about the problems of the current healthcare system, challenges with current insurance, and the fact that the whole system and approach is broken and now crumbling down. After all, why was homeopathic medicine dropped around the year 1911? Answer: power and greed! "Follow the money," as they say. So, is it easier to buy a car with your own money or collectively as a family where all contribute to the final purchase? I hope you answered collectively, because that is the essence of health cost sharing. The CareXchange community contributes to a shared "pool" in order to cover fees associated with medical costs. Here's an example: rather than paying an average annual health insurance cost of $7,620 for an Affordable Care Act (ACA) marketplace plan, which may only cover certain items, or $8,951 for single coverage, and $25,572 for family coverage, let's say you pay $300 per month into the community, which is more than 50% that of healthcare insurance, right? Now, that $300 gets combined with every other participant's $300. If there is a sudden emergency, such as a heart attack or someone in the family breaks a bone, the money can come from the community to share the cost!

Data from the National Health and Nutrition Examination Survey (NHANES) revealed that as many as 38% of adults and 12% of children have used an integrated medical approach at some point with more than 50% of adults having used at least one dietary supplement in the past 30 days (Millstine, 2023). There is a paradigm shift occurring, a revolution in the realization and need for a better way. Medicare plus Medicaid plus private insurance is not working well, while consuming almost 20% of GDP. Many patients are still not covered by health insurance, while a key trust fund supporting an exorbitant Medicare program has a new insolvency date estimated at year 2036. Does anyone even realize how much it costs to deliver patient care and to what extent do these costs even relate to measurable outcomes? Costs are compiled, scrubbed and analyzed at the specialty or service department level but the overall health picture is lost.

Take a moment and consider the philosophy of CareXchange; The secret sauce, if you will. How we view our lives is fundamentally important. There are two roads: the healthy road and the unhealthy road. Is that the same as "good" and "evil?" That is one way to look at it. The other is living the life we were meant to live. But, "I have a good job," you may say, and, "I'm doing just fine." But ask yourself a few important questions: "Am I stressed? Have I been diagnosed with a chronic illness? Am I taking medication? Do I exercise enough? Do I know how to exercise properly? Am I eating the right foods? Am I taking time for my emotional, physical, and spiritual well-being? Is God important to me? How many true friends are in my circle? Am

I happy?" If any of the above answers are "No," we would suggest making a change. Just one to start. The first one is usually the hardest, then somehow the journey gets easier. Remember, awareness is key and we get to where we are going faster if we know where we are going.

Visualize who you want to become, and how you want to do it. Write down what you feel you need to be happy and healthy. Writing things down is important for goal setting—somehow when things are written down it sounds a call to action to both you and the universe around you. Don't skip this step! Treat your body as a temple. Learn to read labels. Avoid fast food, hydrogenated, super-sized, excessive calorie diets with no nutritional value and remember, if you cannot pronounce the unknown chemical ingredients don't buy the product. If alcohol or smoking is a problem, change the behavior, seek counsel where needed and replace the urge with something else reading, writing, listening to music, playing an instrument, knitting, painting. We can never undervalue the importance of human engagement— talk to a 'buddy' about your quest for change. Who knows, they may have the same issue and need just as much support or even more. Do you agree it's easier to accomplish a goal with the support of another?

We become what we think about, right? So why not take the CareXchange challenge? Test yourself for 30 days—read the ingredients on labels, and don't buy anything you cannot pronounce. Moreover, know where your food comes from. Choosing locally grown organic vegetables and fruits, exercise, walking and praying can lead to happiness. Do your very best to change your perspective(s) and move the dial on your life. Remember, you are not alone on this journey. The power of God is full of wisdom, energy, understanding, and guidance. This is CareXchange: sharing the burden of healthcare costs + coming together in God's name + inspiring a natural, integrated approach to caring for ourselves. ⊶ What positive virtue is gained by looking beyond the traditional healthcare system to include integrated alternative solutions, nutrition, exercise, and spiritual well-being?

Although alternative medicine dates back thousands of years, one key difference as compared to mainstream medicine is the strength of evidence supporting best practices. When possible, allopathic medicine bases its practices only on the most conclusive scientific evidence consisting of double-blinded, randomized clinical trials. In contrast, alternative therapies, because of lack of funding and the organized approaches of the pharmaceutical industry, base their practices on evidence-informed practices. Yet, there is considerable information contained in peer-reviewed publications and textbooks, evidence-based assessments, and expert panel discussions. Therefore, we wanted to take an opportunity to dig a bit deeper into specific case studies and areas of alternative medicine which are quite interesting. "We are Not a Diagnosis!"

CHAPTER 7:

CASE STUDIES

Root of Disease

Let's look at a few examples of how alternative therapies can be of benefit. Dr. Ryke Geerd Hamer, MD looks at the human being in terms of psychic roots of diseases. He discovered the "Five Biological Laws of Nature" which represents a change in the understanding of what is commonly called a disease. Dr. Hamer, through his research, came to the conclusion that the disease processes are not "errors of nature," but, rather, significant biological programs of nature stemming from conflicts such as dramatic events (Taddei, 2012). His theories do not apply to injuries caused by accidents, or poisoning, (e.g. fluorine, mercury, glyphosate, antibiotic pesticides).

What is a biological conflict? "Cancer does not begin in the body—cancer begins in the brain!" A biological conflict is a very primal response to an event in a person's life that completely catches them off guard. These events can be described as a feeling like being struck by lightning. As a result, we develop cold hands and feet, lose appetite, can't sleep, while the mind keeps dwelling on the trauma and making it difficult to want to talk to anybody about it with a "flight-or-fight" mindset. These conflicts, in order to qualify as biological in nature, must be unanticipated and can involve a separation from a loved one, a territorial loss, a self-devaluation, a profound fear, a fight over something that we believe rightfully belongs to us, injuries inflicted through accidents, harsh words, or even a fear for our lives or the life of a loved one. The list goes on, as these biological responses are preprogrammed into our brains, and are responsible for creating most of the disease states we are familiar with today. And "spontaneous remissions" occur when the patient's biological conflict situation finally gets resolved, whether naturally as life changes and adaptation occurs, or after significant conscious effort. Dr. Hamer's theory addresses the "root cause" of disease states. His personal journey with cancer began with a profound emotional trauma. In 1978, his son, Dirk, was murdered in a random act of violence. Three months after this tragic event, Dr. Hamer was diagnosed with testicular cancer. This experience prompted him to explore the connection between emotional trauma and the development of cancer.

Driven by his own experience and the desire to understand the underlying causes of cancer, Dr. Hamer began to investigate the backgrounds and personal histories of his cancer patients. He found that each patient had experienced a severe emotional shock or conflict before developing cancer, which he believed were the triggers for cancer development.

ELECTRIC PULSING:

It is no secret that high frequency electric pulses impact muscle contractions. But here, we are not talking about an electric shock which many of us have experienced where we "jerk" our hands or bodies away from the shock in self-protection and defense. Rather, high frequencies have been demonstrated to aid as an "anti-muter" effect in patients as a potential use in clinical electro chemotherapy. Tumor response was investigated, and included head and neck squamous cell carcinoma, basal cell carcinoma, melanoma, and adenocarcinomas. Combined therapy of application of electric pulses to a tumor, following intravenous or intertumoral drug injection, resulted in objective response rates of the tumors ranging from 62% to 100% indicating that nanosecond pulsed electric fields may influence the permeability of cellular membranes and trigger nonthermal cell death by apoptosis, aid in inhibiting tumor growth, and target intracellular organelles. Frequency dependent pulses of increased amplitude have demonstrated progressive reduction of tumor blood flow with a corresponding increase in tumor cytotoxicity as measured by growth delay indicating that blood flow reduction induced by electric pulses could have future potential in exploiting modalities mediated by tumor hypoxia.

HERBAL THERAPIES:

Cancer:

There are currently over 300 anti-cancer drugs, many of which were extracted or based on natural products or mimetics. However, while pharma recognizes certain bio metabolic pathways, the full understanding of how these natural elements work is still relatively unknown. While single receptors have been shown in science to have an effect when activated or inhibited, the full physiological picture remains unknown and undiscovered. A multinational survey found that 35.9% of cancer patients were either past or present users of complementary and alternative medicine (CAM). Herbal medicines were by far the most used group of treatments, escalating in use from 5.3% before the diagnosis of cancer to 13.9% after the diagnosis of cancer. Mistletoe extracts, particularly from European mistletoe (Viscum album), are used for a variety of conditions including cancer, HIV, seizures, and degenerative joint disease. A review of 18 clinical trials (6,800 participants) demonstrated that "mistletoe therapy" seems safe and beneficial for QoL in adult patients with solid tumors. But there is an urgent need to confirm its efficacy in patient-centered care in a complex oncological setting.

Additionally, scientists have discovered that some other plant compounds can be powerful cancer treatments. For example, drugs like vinblastine, vincristine, topotecan, irinotecan, etoposide, and paclitaxel (Taxol) all come from plants. New plant-based drugs are also being developed to target specific parts of cancer cells (e.g. flavopiridol and combretastatin A4 phosphate).

Diabetes:

One of the most famous examples of an approved antidiabetic drug that was developed from an herb, with a long history of use for diabetes, is metformin, which is derived from the lilac (Galega officinalis). The incidence of Type 2 Diabetes in the adolescent population has increased dramatically despite advances in pharma. Yet, case studies continue to reveal the benefits of an integrated approach, such as in a 12-year-old child diagnosed with T2DM one month prior to visiting a clinic who reported undergoing no pharmacologic treatment. Chinese herbs were initiated and included decoction, Berberine hydrochloride, in addition to physical exercise and diet control, the patient's fasting blood glucose decreased from 8.3 mmol/L to 5.5 mmol/L. Additionally, glycated hemoglobin decreased from 12.9% to 6.1%, indicating that without any Western medicine intervention, his diabetes has been reversed after six months of treatment.

LED/LLLT THERAPY:

Due to a lot of work done by Ron Ignatius dating back to the 1980's, it's now thought that red and infrared wavelengths are absorbed by cytochrome C oxidase, which is a key enzyme in cellular metabolism triggering a cascading feedback within the cell. Altering cellular function using low level, non-thermal LED light is called photobiomodulation (PMB), or low-level light therapy (LLLT), and is a medical treatment modality of increasing clinical importance, as well as red light therapy for the improvement of diabetic leg ulceration, which can be devastating for patients. Furthermore, the influence of LLLT on fibroblast and myofibroblast growth and differentiation is well established.

Music Therapy:

Music therapy often exerts a beneficial effect on many neurological diseases including neuropsychiatric disorders, chronic neurodegenerative diseases, epilepsy, and acute brain injury. Clinical studies have suggested that music therapy can effectively improve patients' dysphagia post stroke. A clinical study enrolled six stroke patients with mixed dysarthria. All patients underwent individual music therapy sessions. The duration of each session was 30 minutes, and 12 sessions in total were conducted. The maximum phonation time, fundamental frequency, average intensity, and sequential motion rates were increased after music therapy, indicating that music therapy can improve speech motor coordination, including respiration, phonation, articulation, resonance, and prosody.

BIOENERGETICS:

Multiple neurodegenerative diseases show bioenergetics dysfunction. With some of the most common neurodegenerative diseases, mitochondrial-related bioenergetics dysfunction could represent a relatively upstream or downstream pathology. The mitochondria is an element of the human cell that contains an "electron transport chain"which ultimately drives the production of energy known as adenosine triphosphate (ATP) which is how we survive. The ATP allows for critical life dependent movement sodium (Na^+) and potassium (K^+) ions across the cell membrane. Bioenergetics flux manipulation may contribute more to Alzheimer's disease management than we currently suspect (Swerdlow, 2014). AD therapy typically includes AChE inhibitor (AChEI) drugs that increase brain Ach levels. AChEIs typically yield modest but noticeable benefits. Remember, the "flux capacitator" in the Back to the Future movie? Imagine manipulating energy frequencies to combat current disease and illness. It has existed for many years in different countries, but has not been explored to its highest potential. There are vast energetic possibilities in which we can utilize and the mitochondria referred to above is just one area of bioenergy exploration.

Extremely high frequencies have also been utilized in some cases of epilepsy. Bioresonance has also demonstrated a reduction in the severity of patients facing recurrent depressive disorder with moderate and mild episodes. The electrical complexity of the human body is astonishing with each cell within the body having its own particular electrical parameters to maintain homeostasis. Cell membranes contain lipid bilayers and different minerals create an ionic push/pull that is always in motion in each cell, known as ionic gating which goes on to facilitate movement of particles inside and out of the cell but so much more is possible and unknown.

All these case studies and discussions regarding causes and effects, as well as treatment options, are clear and concise reminders that not only must we maintain an open mind when it comes to our health, but we are the sole architects of the paths we choose to take when it comes to our physical, emotional, and spiritual well-being. Moreover, it is important to realize there are options available to us outside of traditional medicine that have been impactful. The above mentioned areas deserve further study, realizing randomized clinical trials in these areas are unlikely. The table below depicts just a fraction of alternative options available which continue to expand.

"Mind and Body Practices"

"Natural Products"

Nutritional

Medicinal Plants and Other Products (Ingested, Topical, Inhaled, etc.)

Probiotics
Prebiotics
Phytochemicals
Dietary Plants, Herbs, and Spices

Vitamins and Minerals

Dietary Supplements

Essential Nutrients
Food as Medicine
Food and Microbiome Metabolites
Diet and Dietary Patterns

Botanical Drugs

Drugs

Psychological

Mindfulness and Spiritual Practices
Psychotherapy

Mindful Eating

Meditation
Breathing and Relaxation Techniques

Art
Music
Dance

Movement
Education
Yoga
Tai Chi

Physical

Manual Therapies
Heat/Cold

Acupuncture

Light/Electrical/Magnetic Stimulation

Devices

Surgery

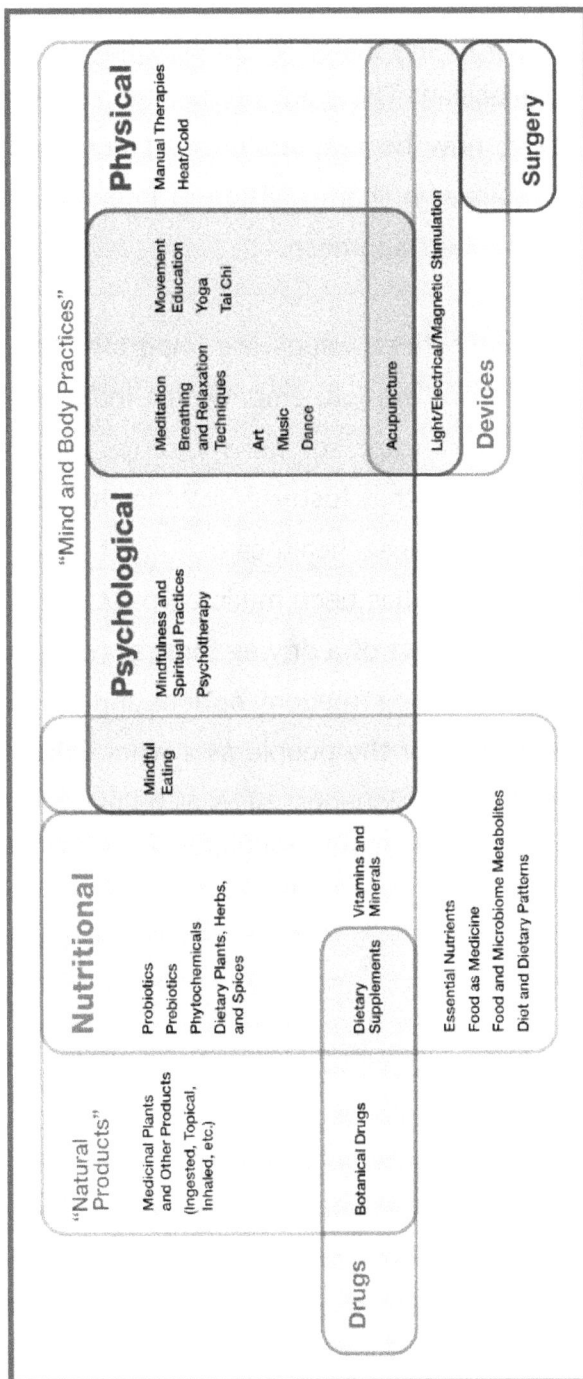

National Center for Complementary and
Integrative Health (https://www.nccih.nih.gov)

Again, CareXchange is health cost sharing, not health insurance. It is a community-driven model that pools monies together for the greater good of each participant. The ability to create your personalized healthcare journey can now be realized through our community of like-minded individuals who share a vision of integrative health through a strength in numbers approach.

We are reminded why these values are important to us and our participants through our mission: empowering individuals with affordable, integrative healthcare solutions through community-driven resources and sharing that foster a healthier future. It may sound simple and it is, because healthcare doesn't have to be complicated. Unfortunately, it has been muddled through the years with pharmaceuticals being part of a driving force that has built an inferior healthcare system lacking freedom, options and alternatives. It is not in the best interest of the people as a whole, nor does it address the individuality and uniqueness of us as human beings and therefore goes against the Oath to which I uphold.

Aside from the financial savings that health cost sharing offers, an open-minded approach to alternative medicine exists, whereby allopathic medicine is not the sole method of treatment. Imagine being able to draw cards from the deck that represent different modalities of treatments, too, and being able to place those cards on the table for inclusion in your healing process. For example, if your preferred treatment is in the homeopathic realm and you'd like to implement a natural path for relief of what ails you, these options may be available, too, along with information that allows for a broader and clearer decision-making process. How about chiropractic or massage therapy to not only alleviate the muscular pain in your back and neck, but also to provide a sense of mental healing through self-care? Yes, yes, and yes! This is an example of holistic healing by taking the whole human being into account when approaching health. Because we are more than the sum of our parts, we must take into consideration the interconnectedness of all of our parts for the whole of us holistically ("wholistically") and how they may feed off each other

The answers are literally in your hands with the click of the mouse and striking of the keyboard. Like we've discussed before, we are all individuals with different backgrounds, beliefs, needs and wants, and what may work for some, may not work for others when it comes to our health; therefore, it's imperative to consider an array of information, which we've done. A "build your own healthy you" feel will come to mind as you continue to engage with our community.

The importance of building partnerships is vital to the betterment of ourselves physically, mentally, emotionally, and spiritually. Building trust is the backbone of any healthy relationship and certainly has become an even taller task after so much broken trust and mistrust can be found within consumer's hearts and minds, as we've been told so many lies. It is time for a disruption in how we care for ourselves and each other. The responsibility can no longer be placed in the hands of those who have exploited their power in their quest for more power and profit. Our only hope is to pull together and reestablish our own community of like-minded, out-of-the-box-thinkers, whose common motives, goals, and values align with our own.

The famous African proverb, "It takes a village" when performing a major task or raising a child speaks to the vitality of community. Furthermore, social factors play into such progress (even digression at times) with regard to reaching one's growth potential, reminding us of the paramount importance of coming together for the benefit of each of us. After all, we are all children of a higher source and "it takes a village" now more than ever!

Before you opened this book and began reading, you did something that you may not have even noticed: you opened your mind. Initially, maybe out of curiosity, but you opened it nonetheless.

Congratulations on achieving the Level 2 milestone!! In the next chapter we will discuss the phenomenon that occurs when we open our mind to something greater and become part of a paradigm shift on our quest to realize the full potential of our body, mind, and spirit.

NOW ENTERING LEVEL 3:

Belief Systems & Transformation

CHAPTER 8:

PARADIGM SHIFT

Any great movement or crusade, for that matter, begins with a shift in thinking. We wrote this book because of a genuine passion for making people aware of such a shift with where things are headed, where they could be headed, and how we can implore others to become part of such a movement, through faith, freedom and shared health care costs. We are living in a time where a paradigm shift is taking place, not only within our healthcare system, but the future of our overall health and well-being is at the precipice of something big. There's so much at stake, and we can either continue to be part of the ever-growing problem or part of the solution. The writing of this book, and you reading it, is powerful evidence that we are choosing the latter! A paradigm shift in the way we think and the way we will take actionable steps in making positive change in our lives, and the lives of others, is in our grasp, and we wholeheartedly believe it can, and will, become a beautiful thing!

Google reminds us that a "paradigm shift" in psychology refers to a *significant change in the dominant theoretical framework or way of thinking within the field, where a new body of evidence disrupts the previously accepted understanding of behavior and mental processes, leading to a new dominant approach. Essentially, a shift from one major perspective to another, like from the behaviorist approach to the cognitive approach* (Oxford University Press, n.d.). There's that word that we love: disrupt! That is the goal here, to disrupt the status quo within the world of health, healthcare, and, more specifically, how it applies to health cost sharing. It takes a profound shift in thinking to disrupt a previous long-conditioned acceptance of something, and we feel a direct obligation to ensure that information is conveyed to as many people as possible in order to increase their quality and longevity of life. This is not about being in the "Sickness" business; rather, it is all about Life Wellness. It is our sincere hope that this book offers you the very new body of evidence that will awaken you to such an important paradigm shift.

Whether it be the Copernican Revolution, which challenged the new idea that the sun was at the center of the universe, yielding the transition from the geocentric model to the heliocentric model, or the shift from Aristotelian physics to the laws of motion and universal gravitation developed by Newton, great shifts in thinking are typically met with resistance. The debate on the Theory of Evolution can still be heard today, and certainly at the time Charles Darwin's theory was considered to be a revolutionary, if not erratic concept. But Darwin's theory invalidates itself as two different species that were to have apparently evolved from one to another cannot coexist. But it does take some shock value to arouse the imagination of society into realizing there is usually more than one theory that can be backed by enough information to get us thinking.

More recently, the Information Revolution has allowed us to do our own research as answers can be found with the click of a computer key. In the world of AI, our world is rapidly changing. Information is at our fingertips and is already infiltrating the medical system. Robotics, statistics, health management, electronic medical records are all "in play" for AI. "Nanorobots" are now being developed for localized and specific medication administration and more. Surgeries can occur from afar with the use of a joystick by a surgeon to operate a robot. But it goes deeper. Currently approved medications are being challenged more by the availability of AI and search engines cross-checking various datasets simultaneously, yielding ever-evolving possibilities for discovery of drug-drug interactions and adverse effects. AI will also avail the discovery of new drug pathways, enhanced physiological and biochemical understanding, and the development of medical robots, as well as new synthetic medications. Smart watches already track heart rate, respiratory rate, wrist temperature, sleep duration, blood oxygen levels and more. Couple this new age of information with the rebellious passion of the 60's and you have a recipe for change that is long overdue within the world of government control, healthcare, and Big Pharma as it applies to our individual health. Yes, we are experiencing a paradigm shift, and the good news is: change is upon us!

Fortunately, we're not alone in our quest to rebel against the world of health's status quo. Ultimately, we must be our own "watch dogs," but if you seek, you shall find many others, too, both on the front lines and behind the scenes, who are on watch when it comes to keeping government, Big Pharma, and regulatory agencies in check for the betterment of our health. Robert F. Kennedy Jr., who now oversees the Department of Health and Human Services, has long been an advocate for freedom of choice through "informed consent." He has made it clear that agencies that have been at odds with mainstream health and science need to return to the gold standard empirically based, evidence-based science and medicine that they were once famous for. Another top priority of Kennedy's is to end the chronic disease epidemic with measurable impacts on a diminishment of chronic disease within two years. He has advised the current administration to remove fluoride from all public water.

Kennedy hopes to reverse the trend of Americans increasingly suffering from a range of acute and chronic conditions over recent decades. Despite the massive amounts of appropriated funds and the tireless efforts of many individuals within the healthcare field, these chronic conditions are on the rise, and Robert F. Kennedy is prepared to get to the bottom of this while pushing to reform policies and restoring compromised government oversight. We definitely are not alone in our belief that the allowance of pesticides and chemicals in our food and skincare products by our own government is compromising our health and quality of life. Moreover, the root cause behind such allowances, again, is money! Kennedy's mission to "Make America Healthy Again" will help to continue a trend of paradigm shifts, while opening the eyes of many that monetary interests and political corruption are part of the root cause of allowing these chronic conditions to continue affecting our nation, while advocating an overall awareness and responsibility of doing our due diligence.

Mike Adams is known as the "Health Ranger" and is another watchdog and advocate for change within the healthcare world. Mr. Adams promotes the idea of putting medical freedom back into the hands of the people. After all, who has the most to gain or lose when it comes to our personal health and the choices we make? We do, of course! So it only makes sense that the decisions to be made regarding our health align with the promotion and availability of alternatives. The "Health Ranger" continues to voice his opinion through blogs and articles which call for a stoppage of criminalizing naturopaths and herbal medicine practitioners. He says, "When Big Government runs Big Medicine, it's complicit with Big Pharma's profiteering agenda that requires keeping people with disease and suffering. Socializing medicine only means making the monopoly, fraud, waste and abuse even worse!"(Adams, 2016).

While both Robert F. Kennedy Jr. and Mike Adams are speaking out against Big Pharma, healthcare insurers, and government agencies putting us consumers in harm's way, we must continue our own paradigm shift of thinking and acting on our own behalf in order to experience a very personal and prosperous outcome. Ultimately, we must be our own watchdogs when it comes to our health and well-being, but it sure helps to know we are not alone. Part of the shift we are discussing is the disruptor mentality, whereby it is no longer acceptable to sit and watch from the sidelines as Big Pharma, large healthcare insurers and government agencies like the FDA dictate what we eat, how we eat, how we care for ourselves and our loved ones, and how we will pay for it all. It has become blatantly obvious that our quality of life should not be in the hands of those with such insidious ulterior motives. We will not be bullied any longer!

Any movement or shift requires a firm belief in the cause and one can find answers as long as they have their eyes open. The evidence is all around with regard to the downward trend in our health as a nation. We talk about the root cause in the medical field a lot, and in this book, we've mentioned it several times because, in essence, we should find the root cause of any problem or challenge we are striving to remedy.

Unfortunately, there has been another shift/trend to allow a Pharma-controlled government to silence your doctor and dictate basic components of your medical care. An example of this effort to relinquish doctor and patient control can be found within an article by Dr. Joseph Mercola, where he outlines the 2023 Omnibus Appropriations Bill which included 19 lines that proposed increased power to the U.S. Food and Drug Administration in their effort to ban off-label use of approved medications. This potentially limits doctors' abilities to freely treat patients, and patients' ability to use all available treatments after making an informed decision (Mercola, 2023). The amendment puts the FDA, and by proxy Big Pharma, at the helm of powerful health care decisions that should be made on an individual, personalized level between a patient and their health care provider. In California, law AB 2098, which went into effect January 1, 2023, gives the state power to take away doctors' medical licenses if they spread "misinformation" that goes against the standard rhetoric.

The FDA is seeking more control over medical practices, which could undermine the physician-patient relationship and medical innovation. This follows a 2021 legal ruling that limited the FDA's power to interfere with medical practices. Furthermore, the FDA's

THE LIFE WELLNESS COLLECTIVE

funding from the pharmaceutical industry raises concerns about bias and the influence of Big Pharma on medical decisions. Again, "follow the money," and you will find the root cause of why such decisions are being made in a manner which is entirely counter to our best interest. Who benefits most from this shift in power? The answer is plain to see, and our voices have been subdued far too long. We have been sold a false bill of goods when it comes to our own health and well-being, and we have found ourselves in a unique time in our history where the stakes have never been greater; the ideas we've been force fed are much more transparent than ever before, and this notion, coupled with our empowered sense of self free-thinking, puts us in a position to be at the forefront of our own paradigm shift.

We have an obligation to ourselves and those we love to shake things up for the future of our society. Disruptors in the greatest sense, with purpose, by taking our health back into our grasp and ensuring ourselves as whole-hearted human beings, not only to live the best life we can, but to make sure that the eyes of future generations are wide open. Health cost sharing is certainly part of this shift, and we believe CareXchange is a giant step in the right direction, as it was created with a core belief that we are worthy of the best possible options when it comes to our own quality of life. After all, if we don't believe we are worthy of the very best options when it comes to our health, who else will? The world is changing, and the time has never been more perfect to shake things up and be part of something revolutionary and become the shepherds and not the sheep.

The proverb, "The longest journey begins with a single step," comes to mind when we are talking about disrupting a system or creating a shift in a new direction. That small pebble seems harmless without force behind it but with momentum added, it becomes something incredibly powerful and noticeable. That small ripple in the ocean eventually becomes a wave. We can increase that power when we decide to work together for the greater good. In addition to all the information and technology available to us at the tip of our fingers, we can also benefit greatly by looking back at the simplistic beginnings of how some concepts and movements were implemented. Let's look together at the history of health cost sharing in chapter 9.

Hint: As we assess today's models of care, what belief are you ready to release in favor of healing?

THE LIFE WELLNESS COLLECTIVE

CHAPTER 9.

THE HISTORY OF HEALTH COST SHARING

"When you are surrounded by people who share a passionate commitment around a common purpose, anything is possible."

–Howard Schultz (Schultz, 2016).

The World Health Organization defines "health" as a state of complete physical, mental, and social well-being, and not merely the absence of disease or infirmity." The whole concept of health dates back many years, and its meaning is subjective. Interestingly, the first Oxford dictionary included the soundness of mind, body, and spirit. It is not merely "the absence of disease" aspect of the definition that is intriguing, as this opens the door for multi-factorial components of health–physical, mental, spiritual, social, professional, and financial, which may be influenced by exercise, thoughts, emotion, prayer, and the environment, but what we can do to enhance our quality of life can be equally thought-provoking.

This multi-factorial approach to health dates back to Hippocrates. Yet, if this idea of health has been around for such a long time, isn't there a duty or responsibility that goes along with it? After all, how can we deny that within the very word of health, there is "heal?" Are we healing or masking symptoms? The sense of responsibility of survival is innate in a community. Just look at the animals and their habits for proof. Observe how ants, bees, birds, and even fish work together to achieve goals. The geese fly in V-formation to establish leadership, streamline, draft and guide the misled. For this reason, I would define health cost sharing as instinctual and, therefore, a law of nature. The innate sense within all of us to help each other and come together during challenging times. This is not revolutionary as much as it is common sense because we have a natural tendency to do this in order to achieve goals.

The concept of health cost sharing is not new, as it dates to ancient times in Chinese, Indian, and Greek practices, whereby the need for a balanced mind, body, and soul created the ability to overcome "disease." Recall that bloodletting was used in medicine for over 3000 years starting with ancient Egypt, Greece, and Rome, and continuing into the Renaissance! During the Middle-Ages when there was no such things as insurance workers, different workers, trades, and crafts united to form groups or "Guilds." Then, they would pool resources together, resulting in the groundwork for health cost sharing. Let's take a deeper dive into the history and development of health cost sharing.

The Mennonites are named after Menno Simons (1496-1561), who was a priest in Holland, and read the writings of Martin

THE LIFE WELLNESS COLLECTIVE

Luther, but eventually left the Catholic Church in 1537 and became an Anabaptist preacher and writer. The Anabaptists were Christians who rejected infant baptism and worshiped together in their homes. Similarly, the Amish are named after Jakob Ammann (1644-after 1712), an Anabaptist preacher born in Switzerland. The Amish are conservative Protestants who appeared around 1693. The Amish split from the larger Anabaptist Mennonites and immigrated to America in the 17th and 18th centuries. Many of the Mennonites, as well as the Amish, are against any form of insurance: they rejected it because they felt it placed trust on the world, rather than embracing faith in God's divine promises. Therefore, the church encouraged one another to come together financially in times of need – a concept rooted deeply in Anabaptist history.

There were also fraternal organizations such as the Masons, which formed its first Grand Lodge in London in 1717, and the Knights of Columbus which formed in 1882 in Connecticut to provide support for working-class and immigrant Catholics in the United States. These fraternal groups provided financial assistance and other aid inclusive of health cost sharing. Today, across the United States, there are a whopping 20,000 fraternal benefits associations (Smith, 2023), offering a variety of benefits to their participants, including insurance, financial assistance, education, scholarships, and social activities.

To put things in perspective, during the Industrial Revolution which occurred in the mid-18th century, and again into the 20th century, European society was evolving, growing, and developing with massive innovations, and forcing immigration across the Atlantic in hope of a better life. With this migration came the unfortunate circumstances of poverty, discrimination, language, and cultural barriers. As a result, immigrants began to form "mutual aid" alliances or groups to assist their community, meaning their resources were pooled to aid the sick and needy.

While our founding fathers were drafting the pages of the United States Constitution, the Free African Society, founded in 1787 made available assistance and aid within their circles during times of racism and exclusion–unfortunately, not much has changed in that regard. Let's not forget past mutual aid organizations such as the Knights of Labor, the Farmers' Alliance, and the National Association for the Advancement of Colored People (NAACP), which helped to set the stage for health cost sharing.

In 1892, after migrating to Ellis Island, Jewish workers came together on New York's Lower East Side and formed their own mutual aid society: the Workingmen's Circle or "Arbeter Ring." At this period of time, this group was overworked in what was referred to as "sweatshops," with long hours and no benefits–a virtual slave to the trade. Who would have thought that this group would grow to over 80,000 participants by 1920, providing benefits to immigrants for their health, sickness, and even death/funerals?

Skipping to the arrival of the Great Depression and WWII, we acknowledge hard times, and some participants of the Mennonite community wished to see a formal, church-wide form of aid to help church participants in times of need. This resulted in Mennonite Mutual Aid (MMA), and as the insurance industry developed and grew in the United States, so did the MMA. I recently had a brief discussion with an Amish man who spoke of some of the difficulties of current health cost sharing efforts which have resulted in substantial debt secondary to the exorbitant fees charged by the current healthcare system.

The 20th century saw mutual aid take a central role in the struggle for civil rights and social justice. During the Great Depression, mutual aid networks were crucial for survival, particularly in African American communities that were disproportionately affected by economic hardships. The Black Panther Party "survival programs" in the 1960s which included free breakfast for children, health clinics, and educational initiatives, exemplified mutual aid as a form of resistance and empowerment (Heathcott, 2003). The significance of mutual aid organizations is undeniable in their role in improving the lives of millions of Americans, while playing an additional role in raising awareness of social issues and driving change, while helping the community at the same time.

It is also important to keep in mind the transition occurring in healthcare throughout the years. The 1950s brought the "planning movement" in response to pressures on urban hospitals resulting from suburbanization and the public concerns about rising costs. Healthcare insurance payers like Blue Cross were reimbursing hospitals for depreciation–the system was failing. Continuing through the Reagan years in the 1980s, health planning remained a consistent theme of American health policy. It was at this time that many of the charitable community-based health systems inclusive of Catholic-based hospitals such as St. Joseph's, were challenged financially and forced to close their doors to larger financially rich for-profit hospital systems (Milbank, 2006). The suburban hospitals that resulted from these moves fostered relationships with voluntary health insurance, public policy, research and development, technology and training.

Specialty areas in medicine evolved along with capitalization and profits, enabling modern services independent of race, creed, or religious perspectives. Large, urban hospitals were big money and maintained federal support while offering sophisticated hi-tech services. In 1966, a declaration of purpose from the government stated: "Fulfillment of our National purpose depends on promoting and assuring the highest level of health attainable for every person ... this goal depends on ... partnership, involving close intergovernmental collaboration, official and voluntary efforts and participation of individuals and organizations; [and] Federal financial assistance must ... support the marshaling of all health resources—national, State, and local—to assure comprehensive health services of high quality for every person." (U.S. House 1966b, 9; cf. Cohen 1966, 40)

By the 1970s when President Carter took office, the planning movement was experiencing difficulty due to continued cost escalation and cross-party politics – sound familiar? By the 1980s and 90s, insurance payers and philanthropists began to fade from local communities, taking a more formal and positioned role. We remember how America comes together in times of need. Think about how Hurricane Katrina saturated the south in 2005, Hurricane Sandy in 2012 rocked the east coast, tornadoes wiped out the Midwest in 2013, Hurricane Helene waterlogged North Carolina in 2024, the horrendous California fire(s) in 2025–and how people tried to help.

Does it always have to be a catastrophe to get people to help one another? That is the question!

These natural disasters and even the COVID-19 pandemic highlight the lack of knowledge and unpreparedness of government responses and how communities are left to unite and lend a hand, lift a shovel, feed the needy, deliver medical supplies, provide aid, and help to rebuild. Realizing the state and federal government are failing to stand up for proper, just, and equal healthcare in this unprecedented health crisis, it is time for change.

While health cost sharing kicked off in the ancient times, and with the Progressive Era and immigration of Mennonites and Amish, today most health care sharing ministries are Christian-based organizations, with more modern health cost sharing concepts beginning to appear. The Affordable Care Act (ACA) aka "Obama Care" led by President Barack Obama granted specific exemptions to health care sharing ministries, which allowed them to operate independently and without penalty as long as the rules were followed. What rules, you ask?--Answer: they cannot function as healthcare insurance. Since Obama Care, participation in health cost sharing ministries in America has catapulted to approximately 1.8 million participants at the end of 2024, and is growing (Hawryluk, 2023). This is up from approximately 100,000 in 2010. Why? The realization of a broken system–exorbitant costs have taken over, along with the manipulated behavior noted in today's medical practices. Young adults, especially, are coming to terms with a disturbed medical system and the need to incorporate and align with faith based, spiritual, and religious beliefs while not sacrificing the quality of care.

⊶ What concept transforms health from a transaction into a shared act of care and giving?

Health cost sharing has evolved from years past to community based, and now into a more formalized system which is demonstrating significant growth and development and a credible alternative to a challenged healthcare insurance system drowned by the influences of big pharma and modern science. However, it is far from critique. Rules regarding HSCMs as specified by Obama Care are outlined in Section 1501/5000A (d) (2) (B). It is important to note that exemptions from the individual mandates are no longer necessary—why? Because the penalty for not having insurance coverage was reduced to zero by the Affordable Care Act, in most states. Health cost sharing is still maturing, and further development is needed to achieve a more balanced, sophisticated approach to absorbing costs to achieve better health outcomes.

While things have changed over the years, the one thing that remains constant; there is one God, one body, created in a Divine Universe in which right oversees wrong. Our bodies are spiritual beings, and our worlds should reflect nothing less. Our strength, our power, our health, our finances, our passions, our accomplishments are a gift from the most powerful God. So, health cost sharing becomes simple—caring for each other along the way. Are you ready to get started? Congratulations on accomplishing Level 3!! In Chapter 10 we will delve into one of the greatest ways we can show gratitude for the Godly gifts (our body, mind, spirit) we have been blessed with through self-care.

NOW ENTERING LEVEL 4:

Self & Spiritual Alignment

CHAPTER 10:

SELF-CARE

Thus far we've spoken a great deal about the concept of empowerment and its multi-faceted importance in all aspects of who we are and how we live. Ultimately, our time here on our earthly journey is short, and possibly even a miniscule piece of the overall puzzle. However, through self-empowering choices and actions, we can lengthen not only our time, but also our quality of life, which could, in turn, be living proof to others that they can do the same for themselves. The age-old question of, "Why are we here?" cannot be summed up in one sentence, paragraph, or even book, for that matter. In fact, who is really qualified to even answer such a profound and perplexing question? What if our purpose in this life is to spread love and be good to one another? We'd like to believe this is one of the reasons we walk this earth and share this time together.

Furthermore, one of the greatest examples of this can be initiated through our own self-love. Do you agree that when we love and care for ourselves, we are honoring the very force that created us?

Do you believe that our life is something to behold, cherish, and be thankful for? When we respect our bodies, mind, soul, spirit, and the time that we have been blessed with, we are acknowledging the higher source that made it possible for our miraculous moving parts to work together harmoniously, like the greatest computer system imaginable. It goes well beyond our physical bodies, but this alone should not be taken for granted, and if we take a moment to realize the depth of what it all entails in order for us to breathe, think, act, and speak, all while the perfect computer system within our brain directs us to function in the most amazing way, then maybe we can begin to grasp the very miracle that we are.

With this in mind, we now can act on the very gifts that have been bestowed upon us which may be paid forward to create a victorious cycle of good that is living proof to others, through our own positive energy that we exude, that there is a better way to live. This ideal can be realized in one of the most loving things we can do for ourselves, too, and that is self-care. Self-care truly is self-love, and it is a vital piece of the proverbial puzzle in this lifetime that can be the determining factor of both quantity and quality of our entire life experience. We're not talking about superficial facades which appear only on the surface. Rather, we are looking deeper, by sharing loving acts of nurturing ourselves wholly, both inside and out, while enhancing our overall life experience. Self-care is not a "one-size-fits-all." We have all witnessed someone trying to help someone else who could barely help themselves. Self-care involves different aspects that need to be considered and certainly not limited to healthy lifestyle choices such as food, exercise, avoiding drugs, alcohol and smoking. As well as keeping a regular check on how we feel, our finances and emotions.

Self-care can be a very spiritual experience that is far beyond physical. In fact, the Bible can be a great reminder of the importance of this concept through prayer, seeking solitude, practicing gratitude and kindness, resting, and finding peace, among many other examples. Eastern philosophy addresses the significance of caring for our mind, body, and spirit as a whole in order to provide balance and harmony between our individual selves and our environment. You've probably heard of yin and yang, which is the balance between passive (yin) and active (yang) energies that tap into our own natural resources in order to create our most positive output. Qi is the energy, or life force, that flows through the body. Meridians are the pathways in our body that Qi flows through us. Nourishing our bodies, mind and spirit.

Eastern approaches focus on treating the person, rather than targeting specific symptoms. Self-care and healing cannot be confined to the allopathic system of medicine solely through chemical treatments (pharmaceuticals) because our bodies are more than just one entity. We are spiritual beings, as well, and it is necessary to treat ourselves as such by nourishing the whole of us. There are forces beyond viruses and bacteria that can cause illness, so it only stands to reason that our approach to overall health and well-being must be addressed through a multi-faceted approach which falls under the auspices of self-care. Interesting to note that even definitions like disease and virus have changed over the years: the Latin definition of virus included the words "venom" and "poison" which have long since been removed. Emotional and mental triggers can manifest themselves in the physical form, as well, so it is crucial that we feed our emotions and mental health through self-care. We've spoken a great deal about the importance of the holistic approach to health that focuses on the body, mind, and spirit when it comes to treatment, and that really is a perfect example of self-care.

Dorothea Orem was a leader in self-care and defined it as "the learned and deliberately performed action utilized to regulate development and functioning" which resulted in her Self-Care Deficit Theory (SCDT) where she further elaborated that self-care is a developmental process suggestive of health, life, and well-being (Hartweg, 2015). This further suggests the relationship between humans and their environment. This became evident during Covid-19 where many of us became caregivers while monitoring our own symptoms—every person has the capacity to become a self-care agent and practice self-care activities. This can lead to more comprehensive interactions with healthcare providers, better education, improved independent living, chronic disease management and overall well-being.

Self-care is limitless and encompasses whatever it is that feeds your entire being and brings you joy, yet less than 10% of people in the U.S. engage in any health self-care on an average day. It really encompasses whatever it is that feeds your soul, nourishes your body, mind, spirit and that which brings you joy. Taking a walk outdoors is a simple way to invigorate yourself and get in tune with nature while bringing balance and perspective to your life. Yoga not only improves flexibility, strength, balance, and coordination in a physical sense, but it also reduces stress, improves mood, as well as enhancing focus, concentration, and increased self-awareness. If you live near an ocean or a lake, take advantage of the sounds, sights, and calming effects that a body of water can bring. Hiking near a stream is also a perfect way to get in touch with nature and recalibrate yourself. Even something as simple as journaling is a healing way for reflection and expression. By physically touching the earth by "grounding," or "earthing," we connect to our planet's natural electrical charge which neutralizes positive charges and absorbs electrons, which may possibly impact inflammation, improve sleep, enhance cardiovascular function, and promote overall well-being.

Whether you're practicing a form of relaxation or simply enjoying the peaceful silence under a tree, you can enjoy the healing powers both physically and emotionally. Being mindful, kind, and present speaks to your gratitude and appreciation for this miracle we call life. Self-care embraces the belief that you do, in fact, love yourself, God, and others. Are you realizing your self-worth while providing a living example for others to do the same? Imagine a world where everyone felt a little better about themselves and had a more peaceful, kind spirit; our species would not only look better, feel better, but we would also get along with each other in a more harmonious way, while also extending our quality and quantity of life. "There is but one solution to the intricate riddle of life: to improve ourselves and contribute to the happiness of others." (Shelly, 1823).

We have experienced firsthand the importance of self-care in the capacity of loving ourselves, and how that in turn impacts others. The change in perspective among patients that feel the energy and passion we exude is reciprocal. We receive as much satisfaction from not only the life-enhancing medical information we share, but also the fact that we are affecting others in a positive light. Again, it's about the love and human connection that fulfills needs on all levels. Raising a child or caring for an elderly parent, hugging them, feeding them, and nurturing them, adds not only to their life experience and joy, but it also can add years to their lives. These acts of love that seem simple, habitual, or traditional in nature truly can be transcending among all parties involved. A quote from Ernest Hemingway includes the following passage: "What we yearn for is simply human connection—a quiet presence, a gentle touch. These small gestures are the anchors that hold us steady when life feels like too much."

Allow yourself to experience a healthier and more fulfilling life experience because after all, tomorrow is not promised, and even the small enhancements to our journey can make it that much more fulfilling. Making the decision to integrate one positive change makes some small, positive changes in how you treat yourself, can and will benefit your life, as well as the loved ones in your circle. It's a "win-win," resulting in a living example of inspiration. and you will not only bring more longevity and vitality to your life, but your family, friends and loved ones will benefit from you being the best you that you can be, while serving as a living example of inspiration. Have you already begun or are you ready to kickstart your journey to the most fruitful chapter of your life? You deserve the very best this life has to offer, and it begins with an affirmation of love through self-care.

We are physical and emotional beings and have needs that exceed the basic physiological requirements to sustain life, while living our best life possible. With his timeless contribution to psychology: "Maslow's Hierarchy of Needs," Abraham Maslow emphasizes the importance for us to feel safe and secure, while also fulfilling our esteem needs of belonging, as well as feeling a sense of accomplishment (Maslow, 1943). The ultimate goal of self-actualization whereby we would experience the achievement of our full potential, including creative activities, may seem like a lofty goal to some, but it certainly is possible to at least strive for this, while enjoying the journey along the way with an open heart and open mind. These concepts epitomize the idea of self-care and are a cornerstone of CareXchange.

Is there a connection between self-care and faith? We will further discuss this in chapter 11, particularly how being faithful can bring balance to our lives, thus enhancing our health journey. Whatever your beliefs may be regarding our creation—our bodies, minds, and spirits are indisputably miraculous. This proof alone should inspire us to nourish and nurture ourselves to the best of our ability. However, most of us, to some degree, take this for granted, or simply are too preoccupied to acknowledge this. Taking better care of ourselves isn't just a lifestyle we can implement so that we can bring fulfillment to us alone, but also so that we can share with others the possibilities to do so too, all while honoring God.

🌿Hint: Are you restoring yourself — or simply surviving?

CHAPTER 11

FAITH

Everyone's mind may work differently when it comes to making decisions. We all have past experiences which shape our everyday existence and how we respond to challenges, struggles, questions and choices. It has been historically noted that Benjamin Franklin made a point to write out a list of pros and cons when facing such situations, and this method has certainly stood the test of time. Sitting down with a spouse and/or trusted advisor to discuss what the advantages and disadvantages are, and how they may relate not only to the person making the decision, but also their family, is a powerful way to decide something of importance. We have found that prior to answering the question: "What should I/we do?" the response quickly reveals itself and brings clarity immediately after asking another equally, if not more important question: "What would Jesus do?" (WWJD)?

Prior to moving forward with CareXchange, we did plenty of research on health sharing and found out very quickly that the organizational infrastructure has always been a faith-based one. In fact, Federal law in the United States defines healthcare sharing ministries as non-profit organizations whose members are united by shared religious or ethical beliefs. Unfortunately, the formation of a new health sharing company is impeded by a clause of the Affordable Care Act stating that they should be in existence since 1999. Nonetheless, the fact that the concept of health cost sharing is backed by faith made our decision easy to move forward with our program. The answer to "WWJD?" was obvious to us because CareXchange would align perfectly with the concept of helping others, which is something we have dedicated our lives to doing. Moreover, CareXchange is built on truth, ethics and fairness, while building meaningful healthy relationships.

So, if the mission is faith-based, it drives the question: "What is Faith?" Faith can come in many forms, and we certainly believe that our world would be vastly improved on several levels if everyone respected each other's differences and lived their lives in faith, not only in a higher power, but faith in each other as well. When we write a check, we have faith in the vendor to process the purchase. When we get into our cars, we have faith that the car will start, and if we were in an accident, the airbags would deploy, and we would be safe. We have faith while driving that others in automobiles will also drive on their respective side of the road. Faith is all around us and we have it in many things. Specifically, we're talking about faith not religion here. Moreover, the processes of making important decisions whether it be from our leaders, organizations, or our fellow human beings, would be vastly improved if such thoughtful questions were asked prior to enacting the next move, or action. Outcomes would be influenced by spiritual intent and belief, thus uplifting communities and inspiring the populace.

While our world has progressed, and technological advances such as AI will drive the future, the morality of mankind is still the same. Drug abuse, theft, sexual assault, pornography, political upheaval, and racial differences, just to name a few, continue to be widespread. Is there no hope? Is there fear and hopelessness? The Bible in 1 Corinthians 13:13 speaks of "Faith, Hope and Love, but the greatest of these is Love." This order is important because without faith and belief, how can there be hope, and without faith and hope, how can there be love? The answer lay in knowing the truth. People will "know the truth, and the truth shall set you free!" So, what is the truth? It's all around us in all the wonders we are exposed to every day—marriage, the birth of a child, graduation, a new job, new car. So, is love from God the truth that provides the doorway of faith, love, hope and freedom?

Do you trust, believe and have faith? What do you believe? It reminds me of the story of a man in a flood, and he has climbed to the rooftop to prevent himself from drowning. A rescue boat came by and told him, "Jump in and let me take you to safety." The man responded, "No, God will save me." This occurred again with a helicopter and the man responded in the same way. He later drowned and was met at the pearly gates, and the man asked the Lord, "Why didn't you help me?" The Lord responded with, "I sent you a rescue boat and a helicopter!" Sometimes we do not realize the presence of God when it's right in front of us. This is a massive topic, and such principles lay a moral compass for health cost decision-making. Couldn't our world use more of this? Perhaps the restrictions on health sharing are God-sent because at CareXchange we believe we can do more. Imagine if governments followed these models when creating laws for the very people they are supposed to represent? The landscape of our healthcare system would certainly look and feel different if these values were emulated prior to making the rules.

Faith and spirituality play crucial roles in our overall well-being. People who identify as being spiritual tend to live longer, and suffer less illness, while recovering faster. Those who embrace a faith-based lifestyle also suffer less depression, while cases of substance abuse are less common. As medical professionals, we have both experienced firsthand having to make split-second decisions that saved lives; chest tube insertions, trauma, respiratory and cardiac arrest, shootings, stabbings, drug overdoses, fractured bones, and mental illness, just to name a few. We have seen critical patients with severe lacerations recover, as well as experiencing countless open-heart, brain, and other major surgeries, as well as observing the insertion of the "Cleveland Clinic Nimbus" artificial heart in futuristic research in the 90's. We saw patients in the emergency room who were propelled through the front windshield of a car on impact, thrown twenty yards, and they survived! We have seen patients die who we thought, in our medical opinion, should have lived, while others lived who we thought were going to die. Miracles do occur every single day!

Believing in something beyond ourselves can foster optimism and hope with an attitude that boosts mental and physical health. Spiritual practice such as prayer can reduce stress and anxiety. Our bodies are the vessel in which our souls are housed, while our senses connect to the material world, and our minds include thoughtful consciousness that encompasses our mental lives. Our spirit is our essence, including our soul, which represents our higher existence and ultimate connection to God. We are naturally spirited beings that can tap further into our faith, which will, in turn, offer life-enhancing balance and harmony. All of our synergistic pieces are interconnected contributors to our well-being, and faith can be the very anchor that stabilizes us through good and challenging times. As we discussed in our "History of Health Sharing" chapter, the concept of communities coming together and pooling monies and resources for the sake of helping their neighbor. As well as the betterment of all exemplifies a faith-based network. At the core of its ideals within CareXchange, there exists a commonality of helping one another because it's the right thing to do.

What does faith mean to you? For some, it may mean belief in a God, a higher power, or a way of life. But let's start with the word belief by itself. Do we believe a chair will support our weight when we sit down? We trust a chair before we sit down, right? So, we also trust our doctors, our government, our businesses, our banks, our grocery stores and manufacturers. Where does this aspect of trust start and stop? One might say it doesn't stop. And if that is so, why stop there? How many of us go to bed angry or worried, or nervous, anxious about tomorrow? How many of us toss and turn for hours in thought about a recent fight, break-up, health, illness, finances, tests, meetings, loved ones, and career paths? Through faith, we can leave those concerns and worries outside the bedroom, realizing that we have worked hard and triumphed—while there may have been challenges and upsetting news, the day is complete, and tomorrow is a new day! We can make the choice to start fresh because "If God is for us, who can be against us?" (Romans 8:31): after all, God loves us, and He will support those who believe."

Peace is not achieved by taking medicines, injections, tablets and capsules. Along with allopathic medicine by itself comes bitterness, anger, and fear, especially when things go south and treatments and therapies are not working. A downward spiral of emotion for chronic illness can be devastating. The choice is in your hands.

"We are truly unique," Mark Batterson writes in his book, entitled A Million Little Miracles (Batterson, 2024), reminding us that "a woman carries over one million eggs in her ovaries, yet it takes just one to be fertilized." As we grow and mature, the body replenishes approximately 330 billion cells each day and 37 sextillion biochemical reactions occur within us every second. We have approximately 30 trillion red blood cells, each containing 260 million molecules of hemoglobin carrying oxygen to keep us alive.

Have you ever seen the Grand Canyon on a clear starry night, or a beautiful butterfly illuminated with color? Do you feel the earth as it rotates on its axis? Why is there night and day? Why do we rest? Moreover, why do we dream? To sense this grandiosity is humbling and may make us feel insignificant, yet a bigger part of the storyline— like one prop in a major movie. Does anyone else notice? Perhaps not, but that does not mean we are insignificant. Yet, why are we here? Why do some die and others live? Why are there wars and catastrophes, and why do some achieve wealth, power, and good health, while others are homeless and without food?

Science cannot grasp how significant the body is, nor can it comprehend the cause and effect of all the human reactions occurring simultaneously, it cannot be predictive in fully understanding that one medication may trigger an onslaught of other reactions and side effects. Science cannot grasp the spinning of the earth and how that continues year after year. Oh my, what happens if we build too much on one side of the earth versus another—will it wobble? How can water fall from the sky, and why is every snowflake different from the rest? Science cannot grasp the implications of 5 and 10G phones, and lithium batteries, and the manmade effects on the environment and the landslide of events this is creating, such as hurricane, flooding, tornadoes, temperature changes, food quality, and this includes the impact on health. Our phones are approaching microwave frequencies, yet we put the phone to our ears or use ear buds. Could this be affecting us negatively? It would take less than 30 seconds to find several reports that say it does!

Do you mind if we resonate on the fact that God created mankind in his own image? (Genesis 1:27). Can we realize that there is a purpose, and while we may not understand it, things are already in motion? Is it our duty, our responsibility to live life to its fullest, rather than wondering "what if?" at the end of our days. Or if only? Henry David Thoreau wrote, "The question is not what you look at, but do you trust what you see?" Look beyond–when a pilot lands a plane, he/she does not look immediately in front of the airplane; rather, they look down the runway to better gauge where the plane is positioned, so the pilot can better ensure a safe landing.

Imagine for a moment how complete trust or confidence in someone or something is beneficial to our quality and quantity of life, but it can also restore and strengthen our relationships with each other, while we see things through a faithful lens. As our world currently seems to be moving faster than ever, and new and improved technology allows us to communicate more than ever, maybe we've lost a little of that human connection. Have you looked around and noticed everybody on their phone? Are we sharing any quality time together? When was the last time your family sat at the table together and shared a meal without electronic devices—just talking and listening while providing insights, stories and having a good time together? Have we become consumed in hearing all the noise while missing out on the important stuff? Have we divided as people and gotten caught up in he-said/she-said critique of one another? We like to believe these examples are the exception and not the rule. It certainly couldn't hurt us to slow things down and subscribe to a doctrine that promotes community. Remember, it's all in our perception, and when that's not working—we have the power to change it!

Whether making everyday decisions or, specifically, healthcare choices, equipping yourself through your faith certainly can help you with a guiding light. Decisions backed by faith are most likely to be successful endeavors because they are rooted in goodness. We're not talking about a specific ideology or a religion, but a deep faith in something beyond our material selves. We are a diverse species with so many wonderful differences, yet we share something so dearly in common: we were all created somehow, someway, and we walk this earth together. A shared connection through a higher source has brought us here, and we have proven to do some great things when we work together. ⊙——⇀How do unseen forces support your health journey and deepen your inner trust?"

CareXchange promotes the idea that sharing is indeed caring, and through hard work, research, and prayer, we believe we have created a collective that can make a difference in people's lives. There is not only power in numbers, but when there is a direct alignment of a faith-based connection, a sense of stability and community shines on all those involved. We can all use a little more of that feeling of love and belonging, which can prove to be the greatest medicine ever created.

I feel compelled to call out this short text of declaration found in the desk of a pastor who was martyred in Zimbabwe more than 100 years ago and also credit my brother for mentioning this in one of his sermons:

"I am part of the fellowship of the unashamed. I have Holy Spirit power. The dye has been cast. I have stepped over the line. The decision has been made. I am a disciple of His. I won't look back, let up, slow down, back away or be still. My past is redeemed. My present makes sense. My future is secure. I'm finished with low living, sight walking, small planning, smooth knees, colorless dreams, tamed vision, worldly talking, cheap giving, and dwarfed goals. I no longer need prominence, prosperity, position, promotions, plaudit, or popularity. I don't have the right, first, tops, recognized, praised, regarded or rewarded. I now live by faith, lean on His presence, walk by patience, am uplifted by prayer and labor by power. My pace is set. My gait is fast. My goal is Heaven. My road is narrow. My way, rough. My companions few. My guide is reliable and my mission clear. I cannot be bought, compromised, detoured, lured away, turned back, deluded or delayed. I will not flinch in the face of sacrifice, hesitate in the presence of adversary, negotiate at the table of the enemy, pander at the pool of popularity, or meander in the maze of mediocrity. I won't give up, shut up, let up, until I've stayed up, stared up, prayed up, paid up, and preached up for the cause of Christ. I am a disciple of Jesus. I must go 'til He comes, give 'til I drop, preach 'til all know, and work 'til He stops me. And when He comes for His own, He'll have no problem recognizing me. My banner will be clear!" (Manning, 1996, p. 31).

This text is so impactful, so genuine, it's so alive! This is a force field that we all can have, but we alone are responsible for the effort. We know faith will serve us well as it exists deep within, impacting our body, mind, and spirit. This connection is powerful and intrinsic, but faith alone will not make our decisions for us, as it is necessary that we take the knowledge, experience, and faith of our unique health journey and use what we've learned, and what we will continue to learn. Congratulations on achieving Level 4!! As we will discuss in chapter 12, it is imperative that we continue navigating our own healthy journeys with an open mind and heart to seek and embrace the truth, while implementing positive actions.

NOW ENTERING LEVEL 5:

Connection & Collective Action

CHAPTER 12:

HEALTH JOURNEY
"WELLNESS BEGINS WITH "WE."

"Wellness encompasses a healthy body, a sound mind and a tranquil spirit. Enjoy the journey as you strive for wellness."

-Buddha

How many of us feel sick, have a fever, rash, upset stomach, muscle ache, back pain, headache or many more countless symptoms and say: "I don't feel well, what do I do?" The conscious mind replies: "I don't know, take an aspirin, an antibiotic, extra vitamin C?" "Well, something has to work, right?" Sometimes, all it takes is one person, one voice, or one message to remind us that we are not alone. People helping people by speaking up and standing up for what is right is a reassuring notion that runs deeper than the spoken word itself. It's about human decency, dignity, and fairness, which should be the rule and not the exception. No human being should be denied the opportunity to have access to the most up-to-date information that can make a difference in one's quality of life. It's ethically and morally wrong. Yet, in a world of misinformation what is the truth? When discussing health and care within the medical world, patient advocacy refers to actions taken to support and protect the interests of patients. Unfortunately, this isn't always the case when we're talking about the current landscape of care. There is a tremendous need for guidance in navigating the healthcare system and what is actually needed and what is not.

Healthcare standards continue to evolve and change and mRNA vaccines and associated delivery platforms, whether good or bad, are becoming the gold standard. At the same time the "Recommended Daily Allowance" (RDA) for vitamins and supplements remains unchanged and only refers to what is needed to prevent serious vitamin deficiencies and not to create maximum health. Therefore, what is the correct amount of vitamins and in what combination? We are not all the same. Many factors need to be addressed to individualize what works and what doesn't include, but not limited to: health state, age, hydration, absorption, exercise, social habits, and more.

While we are discussing standards, also realize that acceptable cholesterol levels used by the medical field was significantly higher in years past and now the levels are pushed so low that testosterone production gets inhibited. So, what is super popular right now— testosterone injections. Healthcare can be a confusing road to navigate, but oftentimes it is paved with high costs, contradictions, and processes that run counter to overall wellbeing. When we don't have the answers we need, who shall we turn to? Moreover, when the very government entrusted to aid in ensuring adequate healthcare and correct information and options for healthy living is failing us, who can we trust to help guide us in making the best choices for ourselves and our loved ones?

Individuals need guidance on their journey for health to ensure proper decision-making to feel empowered and informed. How many people, once diagnosed, go online and download multiple pages of information to learn what is happening and how to fix it? Does that mean they know what to do? Does the healthcare team know, for that matter? Recently, we became aware of a ninety-nine year old relative who was temporarily placed in skilled care for painful shingles, and was literally quarantined like a prisoner and blocked from other human contact because the staff failed to understand how the illness spread. Nobody could approach him unless they gowned in Hazmat equivalent Zoot suits. There he was, dosed with Tramadol which did nothing but mess with his brain, and he started to deteriorate quickly. If it weren't for family intervention, removing unnecessary medications and restoring his independence, he would surely have perished.

Despite scientific papers dispelling erroneous facility policies, the facility refused to acknowledge or change their policies despite the fact they were built on fear rather than the truth. How many of you have your own war stories? Kauffman, Tress and Sherry examined trends over time in medicalization of children with Amplified Musculoskeletal Pain Syndrome (AMPS), whereby a medical record review of 899 subjects ages 3-20 quickly identified a trend of increasing medicalization which introduced risk of iatrogenic injury, and burdened families with unnecessary medical costs. The significant increase in medicalization of children with AMPS is not related to an increase in patient reported pain, which is evidenced by the lack of change in patients' pain score, or pain duration. Then why were these medications continuing to be increased if they were not helping? This has become a pattern which is still a significant issue, not to mention drug-drug interactions, which often go unchecked leaving practitioners to chase and treat symptoms as opposed to root cause.

It's one thing for the average person who may have access, resources, and time to search for answers when they are not initially given, or they are unclear either by communication, or by their own devices, but it's something altogether different for those who are less fortunate or do not understand how to navigate the complexities of the healthcare system. Beyond the level of disappointment and frustration, lies a single mother, an elderly person, a disabled veteran, or even an individual who is ill but can't afford the proper care. Who's going to help them? Who has the time? Who has the answers? Where do we begin? Who will stand up for those who can't stand up for themselves? If the system is not challenged it will never evolve. These are questions we shouldn't have to ask, but we must if we are ever going to get the answers that are not only needed, but deserved! Yes, our system may be broken, but this doesn't mean we can't find some semblance of clarity and peace of mind. Moreover, we have the right to question and/or get a second opinion, which can be life-saving.

A clear process of coordinating care between healthcare providers needs to be in place, as well. Also, advocating for patients' preferences and concerns to healthcare providers cannot be overlooked or taken lightly as we're talking about much more than just the simple filling of prescriptions and chemical solutions within a human-to -human dynamic that runs deeper than the "Band Aid approach."

Make America Healthy Again channels the unwavering energy of the health freedom movement into a powerful political force for change. Founded by senior staffers of Robert F. Kennedy, Jr., MAHA is more than just talk, it is a mission statement that will inspire and ignite action by our leaders, organizations and individuals alike. It is a reminder that we are not alone in our basic desire to create a healthy and prosperous life for ourselves and our family, with a focus on better science, better food, clean water and air. The status quo will not be tolerated anymore when it comes to information, expectations, and processes. The healthcare system is teetering on the edge of a financial, quality, and efficacious cliff, which is crumbling due to jammed and unbalanced policies in need of disruption, if it is ever to rebalance.

Secretary of Health and Human Services Robert F. Kennedy Jr. is already making his voice heard as he has vowed to Make America Healthy Again. Politics aside, one thing that is indisputable is that he has taken an advocacy stance for the greater good, to, at the very least, be aware, awake, diligent, and open-minded to alternative approaches to healthier living. The presence of someone like R.F.K., Jr., who is unafraid to speak up and shake things up, may be exactly what is needed to advocate awareness. His focus is to combat chemical pollutants and additives that he claims contribute to chronic disease in the United States.

Mr. Kennedy is known for promoting healthier diets, discouraging seed oils and pesticide-heavy agriculture. He has cited that, "Many ingredients used in U.S. foods are not permitted in European countries." Reiterating that, "The reason for that is corruption." Kennedy, Jr. has been vocal in his stance against placing profits before public health, stating, in his Five Health Policy Stances: "The food industry and big agriculture producers control the FDA, and so they're not worried about public health; they're only concerned about advancing the mercantile interests of those corporations." {AJMC}.

It should be a personal vendetta for all patients to receive safe, efficacious, affordable and quality healthcare. There is little room for the days of extreme medical error, especially given superior monitoring and educational tools for the healthcare profession(s). Patients have a right to privacy and confidentiality and require help to navigate healthcare disputes and complaints. In today's current state, patients and providers need to better understand how to become and stay healthy, while promoting empowerment and self-management of health conditions where possible. If this is not possible, connecting patients with the proper support groups and resources becomes critically important. ⊙—🔧What do we discover along the health journey when we realize we're not meant to heal alone? The Mayo Clinic comments that support groups provide an opportunity to share feelings and concerns, coping strategies, and unite with the comradery and understanding of going through similar illnesses, conditions, diseases and treatments. This may fill a void between medical treatment and the need for continued emotional support.

Education is key to gaining the necessary knowledge to initiate change. The moment you begin questioning the confusing and frustrating systems in place is the moment you begin empowering yourself with the tools to make a difference through action in finding a better way, then sharing that with others. Yes, this requires a degree of due diligence and some gumption. It all begins with an open mind to alternative approaches, while thinking outside of the proverbial box with what we've been fed (pun intended). There can be no greater advocate for yourself than yourself! After all, you have the most to lose when you accept the status quo as the standard.

You can find the answers and maximize the system in place to its full potential, or you can find a better solution altogether where you're not limited to the constraints within a confining space, often by design and/or apathy. We have always felt a direct connection with our patients, and we write these words through our voices to spread the word and the love based on a truthful desire to provide the most educated and helpful care available–we devoted the majority of our lives to this quest.

Hopefully, you will receive many takeaways with this book, but if there's one defining concept we hope to impart to our readers, friends, and family–it is the importance of community, love and belonging. Historically, tribes, groups, and people thrive when they work together for the common good. Wellness begins with "We." There is a direct connection between community and healthy outcomes. Children who are nurtured and feel part of a connected familial system have greater chances of longevity and prosperity, thereby paying it forward through acts of kindness and giving back because of what they were blessed to receive. We are at our very best when we work together within a community setting. We become healthier and happier when we share with others. A simple act of kindness begins as a ripple that evolves into a wave that can be felt oceans away.

Each of our journeys is unique and representative of who we are and what we choose. It isn't difficult to be overwhelmed with the bombardment of information out there. It can be confusing and contradictory at times. Does it have to be complicated? No, it does not! Oftentimes simplicity speaks the loudest. As we move toward chapter 13 of this book, and possibly your next chapter of your health journey, let's get back to the basics with a simple and powerful formula and the science behind CareXchange.

"To know even one life has breathed easier because you have lived; that is to have succeeded."

-Ralph Waldo Emerson

CHAPTER 13

THE CAREXCHANGE FORMULA™

"Quantum healing involves healing the body and mind from a quantum level, which is not manifested at a sensory level, emphasizing that our bodies are ultimately fields of information, intelligence, and energy."

-Deepak Chopra

For decades, we have tried to understand human well-being through models that focus primarily on the physical body, occasionally expanding to include emotional or social influences. Some frameworks go further, acknowledging spirituality or psychological resilience. Yet even the most comprehensive models still leave a gap. They rarely account for the profound ways spiritual growth, personal transformation, and divine influence shape our capacity for healing and wholeness. The CareXchange Formula™ was created to bridge that gap. It integrates the physical, lifestyle, emotional, spiritual, and divine aspects of well-being into one coherent expression. It recognizes what many people intuitively feel—true wellness arises not only from what we do, but from who we are becoming and the divine grace that sustains us. This chapter introduces the CareXchange Formula™, breaks down each component, and explains how the model can help readers understand their own health journey in a deeper, more holistic way.

So, hold onto your hats! You are about to be blown away!! Imagine two different independent systems, or for that matter, two separate particles. Now, let's say that the two particles share some commonalities and, therefore, the same time and space. At this point, each particle is individually in an uncertain state until it is measured, at which time, the other particle's state also becomes uncertain. This paradox represents the linkage or communication between the two particles. This ties to the concept of "entanglement" where widely separated systems can act as a single quantum entity. I know this sounds "different," but go with it for a few minutes. Now there are elementary particles like protons and electrons, and more hypothetical preons, quarks, and leptons. Electrons can only be ionized by light signifying a specific wavelength, and since we have protons and electrons throughout our body, what if we exhibit wavelike energy? Can we emit our own quantum field? The short answer is "Yes," there has been a lot of research on this topic, so we will not delve too deeply into this aspect. Rather, we will emphasize the quantum connection.

The body is a complex energetic system while also being driven by emotion, intellect, love and a relationship with God. Cells in our bodies emit weak pulses of light—a phenomenon known as "ultraweak photon emission" (UPE) or biophotons. In fact, the skin is known to transmit electricity, and wounds are known to alter electric fields. What if through the concept of entanglement there was harmonic resonance, energy, and wavelengths creating a quantum field? Moreover, what if God had a quantum field that transcends the heavens and stretches out like a tent, and what if God was light (Psalm 104:2, Revelation 21;23)? Also, what if God's quanta is entangled with ours? German physicist Werner Heisenberg described an uncertainty principle as the state where we cannot pinpoint the position of an object with arbitrary precision. The more we try, the more unclear it becomes. So how can we pinpoint the position of God? The vastness of the quantum world still baffles scientists and defies the realm of description by mankind. Now, we have heard of electric pulsing, but what if God's energy was pulsing like the heart (think electricity)? Is it possible that a "super-radiant" condition could be established between the two entangled systems, creating an ensemble of excited atoms, molecules, and cells which collectively emit an intense pulse? Is it the presence of God?

Depending on which version you read, the Bible mentions the word heart between 800-1,000 times—should we guard it? (Proverbs 4:23). Perhaps a positive health outcome stems from our heart and life journey. An electrocardiogram (ECG) records the electrical activity of the heart during each heartbeat. An Electroencephalogram (EEG) of the brain reveals different states of consciousness associated brainwave frequencies, of which Theta brainwaves are associated with heightened intuition, relaxation, and a sense of spiritual connection. This is no accident—we are connected to God's life force! And, if incorporated with an integrated health journey, it will lead to strength, recovery, life, and freedom.

These concepts have led us to derive a multidimensional formula herein referred to as the "CareXchange Formula™" that combines elements of health, lifestyle changes, spiritual changes, and divine influence (God's love). To approach it, we'll need to break down the individual components and conceptualize how they could interact within a mathematical framework. Each of these elements contributes to an individual's overall health, and they can be thought of as interconnected components that influence one another. Let's start with a basic premise and build from there. First:

Health = (Baseline health) X (Change)

Now, if we accept that a baseline is needed to ground or anchor any conclusion and create a method for tracking across time and that if change is applied, our overall health can be improved, then we can move to the next step. We can do better than this because there's more! What specifically makes up our baseline health and what kind of change can improve health? And is there something else? Like an 'IT' factor? Let's now take this basis and amplify it:

Introducing the CareXchange Formula™:

Health Effectiveness= (Hb) (Ti) (Gp)

Where **Hb = baseline health, Ti = effect from integrated therapies and Gp = God's presence** AND, if we can accept this then it begs the question what exactly is impacting baseline and what is changing? Therefore, we have to go one step further:

H= (G) (Hb) (A+T+L) (L'+S'+D')

Again, think of it as a multiplication of care and change—where each factor magnifies the others. Where:

*H= Overall health and well-being represents the total experience of health: physical vitality, emotional balance, mental clarity, and spiritual peace.

*G= represents God's constant, sustaining presence — the belief that God holds all things together and gives life at every moment. This presence is always there. It does not change and is the foundation of health, existence and consciousness; therefore, it is constant and set to 1 for mathematical stability. This should not be mistaken for insignificance—it represents the steadying force that keeps every other component from unraveling. Like the laws of physics, God's presence is always there whether or not we acknowledge it.

*Hb= Baseline Health represents how healthy a person is right now, based on their physical condition, habits, and environment. Hb is the starting point on the wellness continuum. Some people begin with robust health; others carry the weight of chronic disease, trauma, or long-standing stress. As an example, this could be assessed via laboratory panels and biomarkers, physical exams, symptom burdens (such as pain, fatigue), clinical judgement, and psychological assessments to name a few. Here Hb becomes the average of each component. Every journey starts somewhere. The CareXchange

Formula^{TM} simply acknowledges that where we begin influences how the remaining factors can work.

*A= Allopathic medical healthcare or conventional medicine includes familiar medical interventions such as diagnostics, medications, surgeries, therapies, vaccines, and evidence-based disease management. Conventional medicine plays a crucial role in treating acute and life-threatening conditions. Yet it is not a perfect system. Some interventions heal; others fall short; many carry side effects or limitations. In the CareXchange Formula^{TM}, 'A' can act positively or negatively depending on the situation.

*T= Alternative therapies include but are not limited to meditation, acupuncture, herbal medicine, chiropractic care, homeopathy, naturopathy, energy healing, and other holistic approaches. People often turn to these therapies for prevention, natural healing, or to address imbalances not fully addressed by conventional approaches. Like 'A', 'T' can vary in effectiveness depending on the individual and the method. It is interesting to note how many people start looking at alternative therapies upon receiving a diagnosis. However, remember you are not a diagnosis.

*L= Current Lifestyle represents everyday behaviors such as diet and hydration, physical activity, sleep patterns, emotional health and stress levels, social support and meaningful connections, substance use (i.e. cigarettes, alcohol, vaping) and work-life balance. Even the best treatments cannot compensate for a lifestyle that works against the body. Lifestyle can be a powerful healing force—or a silent saboteur.

*L'= Lifestyle transformation refers to positive lifestyle changes a person decides to make (e.g. adopting new habits – exercise, sleep, nutrition, sunlight, improving resilience, emotional intelligence, healthier coping mechanisms). Furthermore, L' represents conscious, positive, sustained lifestyle changes that restore overall quality of life. This includes adopting nourishing foods, improving sleep and circadian rhythms, building resilience and emotional intelligence, choosing environments that support peace, learning healthier coping strategies and aligning daily habits with personal values. Transformation is deeper than a quick fix.

*S'= Spiritual growth (e.g. increasing spiritual practices such as prayer, meditation, education, mindfulness, connection to purpose). It is not merely the improvement of character, but the deep inner transformation that comes from walking daily with the Holy Spirit. This growth is nourished through prayer, worship, Scripture meditation, and a life rooted in the presence of God. An exchange of fear for trust, anxiety for peace, resentment for forgiveness, and self-reliance for divine dependence. This transformation radiates outward, influencing emotional stability, physical well-being, relationships, and everyday decisions.

*D'= Divine influence (God's love, grace, faith, spiritual support, divine guidance and intense pulse). Divine Influence is the active grace, love, and guidance of God—the moments of support, clarity, peace, or direction that feel beyond our own effort. Many people describe this influence as healing, inspiring, or transformative. D' reminds us that while human effort matters, it is not the sole source of change. Divine influence can open doors no treatment or habit can open on its own.

Health is influenced and interconnected by numerous factors, lifestyle habits, psychological states, spirituality, personal beliefs and medical treatments. Previous models attempt to capture some of these components, such as the biopsychosocial-spiritual model, but few models fully integrate spiritual and divine dimensions in a measurable, theologically coherent, and mathematically defensible way. This thought process can be implemented now by practitioners of all types because existing models remain conceptual or qualitative, but here we are suggesting a measurable, numeric index that can be tracked over time. While integrative medicine frameworks include spirituality, it has not considered a scalar factor in a formula. This novel approach is the first quantitative, integrative health metric which unifies body, mind and spirit.

We struggled with this CareXchange Formula^{TM} for some time because we thought that from a theological perspective, since God is the constant grounding of all health, life and existence, that 'G' should go in the denominator as the ultimate frame of reference - the foundational, sustaining force behind all healing and well-being and a deep connection to God's love, grace, and guidance. However, while this approach is indeed spiritually correct, if this occurred, the denominator would in essence equal infinity and therefore, the formula blows up mathematically, creating a problem as a practical health index. Therefore, we shifted 'G' to the numerator as we did not wish to lose this perspective.

Subsequently, the resulting CareXchange Formula^{TM} now 'says' that future health depends on where you are right now, what actions you take, and how much you grow or receive spiritual influence. This

119

works for medical doctors and naturopaths because it uses relative deviation from optimal values ('L') such as HbA1c for diabetes, blood pressure, LDL/HDL for cholesterol, glutathione, CoQ10 and intracellular magnesium. This can be expanded to include multiple aspects of health with each getting a score.

While some patients may be young and have no heavenly reason to present at the doctors office with an ailment, others arrive with heaviness because they know that their current condition is a culmination of years of neglect and an unhealthy lifestyle. After all, how far do we get with chronic anger, hatred, depression, sadness, greed, poor nutrition, harmful water quality, and other toxic situations? The medical profession is just beginning to realize the interconnectedness of human emotion and illness.

Imagine the possibilities of how the CareXchange Formula™ can be further applied to consider the negative impact of individual stressors inclusive of electromagnetic influences such as cell-phones, bluetooth and microwaves, as well as environmental stressors, chemical toxins and more. It can further consider desperation versus inspiration as a negative or positive influencer. Lastly, the formula could consider the super radiance or boost of energy from Divine Influence. These layers were intentionally omitted to keep the model practical rather than overwhelming.

The CareXchange Formula™ can be used as an integrated guiding principle for achieving overall well-being, where a person's health is not merely the result of conventional medicine or personal effort alone, but also a reflection of a balanced approach that includes all aspects of care. Combined, these components show that health improves most profoundly when treatment aligns with transformation, when lifestyle improvements meet spiritual growth, and when Divine influence elevates human effort. A person may follow a perfect diet, take the right medication, and receive excellent therapies—yet remain sick if they are trapped in chronic anger, bitterness, fear, resentment, loneliness, or despair. Modern research increasingly confirms what spiritual traditions have long taught: unresolved emotions and spiritual disconnection manifest physically.

The components of the CareXchange Formula^{TM}, inclusive of positioning spiritual and emotional transformation as indispensable, are not optional; rather, they are intertwined parts of healing. Naturally, from a scientific perspective, the CareXchange Formula ^{TM} is a theoretical construct and would need empirical data to validate its assumptions which may prove to be quite challenging but not impossible for any practitioner to begin testing this for themselves!

The CareXchange Formula^{TM} serves as a framework—a way to visualize how multiple dimensions of life and spirit are interconnected and work together to shape human well-being, while reminding us that treatment matters, habits matter, growth matters, emotions matter, and divine connection matters. Most importantly, it shows that healing is a partnership—a collaboration between medical care, lifestyle choices, personal transformation, spiritual growth, and the grace of God. In this way, the CareXchange Formula^{TM} becomes more than mathematics. It becomes an invitation—to see wellness as a sacred, integrated journey in which body, mind, and spirit move together toward wholeness.

The Life Wellness Collective is meant to be a guide to new possibilities, a reminder that you're not alone. Also, a reinforcement of some of the things you may have already known and just needed to hear them again. ⊙—⇥What begins to flourish when we become aware of our condition, accept care, choose change, and trust Divine guidance? Ultimately this book is about choices, community, empowerment, and how wellness begins with each one of us deep down inside and evolves as we choose to evolve through open eyes, open minds, and open hearts. As we enter our final "Wrap Up" chapter let us always remember: We can live a balanced life, even if the landscape around us seems to be going in directions that are counter to wellness. We still have a choice! We can uncover practical tools and holistic approaches that reclaim your health, power and freedom.

CHAPTER 14:

"INSPIRATION OR DESPERATION?"

Hippocrates stated that, "Health is the Greatest Blessing of Life." Hopefully, you have been inspired in your lifetime, and you've learned about a balance between rest, relaxation, stress, and hard work. We all have our moments when we were so engulfed in a situation we couldn't see the forest through the trees. Confusion sets in, followed by frustration and bad judgement. This could be anything—scaling a wall because a wild animal is chasing you is much different than scaling the same wall because it is a challenge and you want to overcome it. One situation is a frantic attempt to survive—"fight or flight," and the other is a determination to conquer a goal. How many parents struggle with the decision-making process around their children, from the time they are born to the time they branch out on their own, get married, buy a house and excel in their job? Every decision takes us on a path and ultimately there is a crossroad point of decision-making, but is it out of inspiration or desperation?

If we can be at peace, we can take so much more in. When we are distressed, it is not optimal for learning or healing. Stick-to-itiveness is important in maintaining good health. Whatever decisions we make at 16 or 18 (i.e., team sports, group activities, music, daily habits) will follow us for the rest of our lives. When things get tough, changing perspective helps—is the glass half full or empty? Developing trusting relationships as compared to being in isolation will also prove fruitful with networking and problem solving. We know of many examples of people who go "quiet" in times of trouble rather than reaching out for help. **Wherever we go, we take us with us.** I visited a patient with congestive heart failure in the intensive care unit—on oxygen and searching for his next breath. He looked at me and said, "I smoked too many cigarettes." If the decision to pick up a cigarette never existed—same or different outcome?

It takes everyday learning and letting go. We are all a work in progress. Peel one layer of change at a time, in your own time. If only we learned stick-to-itiveness earlier! Then, we would all realize the importance of taking care of ourselves. What is one change you are inspired to make? Are you ready for change now? After all, if individuals who have been on a course of self-destruction changed one habit, imagine the difference it would make in quality of life, like the smoker example above. Do you have an "if only?" Is it possible to change it now?

It's not just our bodies that we need to take care of. Our minds also need the same amount of care and attention. We see it as a posture of life to strive for—we can either have good posture or slouch. If we consider implementing all the positive virtues, then we will go about life by doing our best for those virtues which will be in the forefront of our minds, and we will be quick to express them in everything we do. So, whatever is true, what is noble, whatever is right, whatever is pure, whatever is lovely, whatever is admirable—if anything is excellent or praiseworthy—think about such things (Phillippians 4:8). Remember the old song, "You've got to accentuate the positive, and eliminate the negative?" After all, a cheerful heart is good medicine (Proverbs 17:22).

Inspiration exists as we strive to get ahead of our health—to reconnect and reintegrate with nature, and to seek the diving instinct that transcends our being. ⊙—➤What rises within us when we recognize our strength to heal and align with something greater than ourselves? This is not a time to retreat and accept substandard mediocracy; rather, a time for inspiration to search, explore, research, question and consider new medical possibilities, solutions and cures. Some of these may be right in front of us, while some exist in jungles or rainforests, many of which are quickly being lost to development, natural disasters and more. Honor your history and culture and acknowledge moderation without a steady diet of toxic ingredients.

Consider all the resources that are available such as: family and friends, alternative therapies, supplements, exercise, healthy foods, clean air, pure water, music and prayer that can support challenging times. Each person in our circle represents a part of us, so choose your friends wisely. When we appreciate the tremendous gifts of ourselves and our circle of life, health and well-being will succeed. Therefore, embrace them and your journey together. Because no one should walk alone. Together "We Rise!"

Forgiveness is also a powerful tool and leads to healing. Forgiveness of us/ourselves and other people may not always be easy. It is okay to say I was wrong or I'm sorry. It is okay to say I tried and failed. We cannot know true success without failure. What we sow, we reap. Try to be patient with the process. If you plant weeds, they will grow; the soil doesn't care. If you plant seeds, beautiful blooming flowers and healthy vegetables result, so it makes sense to plant seeds in our lives and not weeds. In fact, there is no book about success that doesn't mention failure.

Patients faced with chronic illness and life-threatening challenges fall into more desperate measures and when they engage with healthcare practitioners, a subconscious decision about trust vs. mistrust soon arises—does the provider demonstrate knowledge, are they experienced with my condition? Also, are they vested in "my" care, or more concerned about the "bottom line?" This question may yield challenging and potentially confrontational encounters with the patient-physician relationship. If we can be at peace, we can take so much more in. When we are distressed, it is not optimal for learning or healing. Don't put your life into someone's hands just because he/she is a doctor! Rather, be educated, ask questions, seek solutions and knock at the door of ultimate healing.

While devastating, society at large has a hard time with the concept of death—at what point did it become "unnatural?" Trust is supported from scientific advances, and this very progress has changed the patterns of mortality and causes of death. Modernistic society has lost a connection with the comprehensive intelligence of nature. However, with all the recent medical changes that have occurred, one might argue that upon desperation, the solution no longer lay in "free will" and autonomy, but driven by the coercion of modern practice and the interwoven pressures of what is perceived as acceptable care.

Moreover, it is okay to say no, when we are faced with uncomfortable or unsafe situations, or accept help when needed. When we care for ourselves, we are better equipped to help someone else. In an airplane, prior to taking off, we are always instructed to take the oxygen mask and place it around our mouth to take a breath prior to trying to help others. So, it's true, when we make healthy decisions, the world opens to us, making us ready to help someone else. FEAR can immobilize! However, if we Face Everything And Recover, we can move on. Remember, we are responsible for the effort, not the outcome. If we trust and keep doing the next right thing, help people and give things away, we will receive three-fold back while feeling truly inspired and we will never be alone. Congratulations on mastering Level 5!!

"A generous person will prosper; whoever refreshes others will be refreshed."

-Proverbs 11:25 (NIV)

"Your shadow is a reflection of just who you are; it doesn't change the actions that you make. So do what is right and your shadow will do it, too, because your shadow is a reflection of you."

By David Shearer

NOW ENTERING LEVEL 6:

Integration & Purpose

CHAPTER 15:

WRAP UP

It is not the critic who counts; not the man who points out how the strong man stumbles, or where the doer of deeds could have done better. The credit belongs to the man who is actually in the arena, whose face is marred by dust and sweat and blood; who strives valiantly; who errs, who comes short again and again, because there is no effort without error and shortcoming; but who does actually strive to do the deeds; who knows great enthusiasms, the great devotions; who spends himself in a worthy cause; who at the best knows in the end the triumph of high achievement, and who at the worst, if he fails, at least fails while daring greatly, so that his place shall never be with those cold and timid souls who neither know victory nor defeat." MAN IN THE ARENA SPEECH—Theodore Roosevelt (Roosevelt, 1910)

The healthcare system is broken. Allopathic medicine by itself has gone too far. Don't get me wrong, when it's needed it's needed. But when it's not, it most certainly is not! This is common sense stuff here! But like the saying goes, "Common sense isn't always common." We have more access to information than ever before, and the fact that you are reading this now is an acknowledgement that you are a seeker and a healer. We must believe in ourselves and trust that we have the power to heal from within. That's why an integrative approach is essential because it's about choices, options, and alternatives. While some medications and/or surgery may be deemed essential, others may not. Careful consideration of any medication prescribed should be given. "Do no harm" is an oath that was taken by us Doctors and it continues to be taken very seriously by us. However, if you turn on the TV or look at your computer at all the side effects in drug advertisements, it becomes all too clear that caution must be taken when considering the allopathic-only route.

Have you ever been misdiagnosed? Go on the internet and ask for differential diagnosis for anything and you will get a laundry list of potential illnesses, and while relieving the "symptom," by temporarily lessening the pain—it may not solve the source. Pain medications do not solve root cause—they only mitigate the pain for the moment while in some cases, over-prescribed opioids leads to addiction and opens up an entirely new set of challenges because the root of the problem was never fully addressed.

"But it hurts! I'll do anything to rid myself of the pain!" We've heard this a thousand times. As healthcare providers we want to do as much as possible for patients, but when a system is broken, it does not allow for optimal outcomes. Patients are now questioning the system more than ever, as they should, yet it is unfortunate that navigating their own journey with little insights and assistance, especially while waiting weeks for an office visit in a clinic or medical office that is already over-burdened, has become the rule rather than the exception for many.

We believe we have an obligation to seek more holistic and natural solutions that will maintain our health and achieve this objective extremely effectively and safely while doing this at a lower cost to the patient. Currently, the CDC recommends that by age 18 a child should receive upwards of 18 vaccines, totaling between 76 and 90 doses. Since when did this become an acceptable practice? Was this information fed to us in small doses over the years, making us too trustworthy by those who have been feeding us? What's their motivation? Could it be just to protect us and make us healthier? Or could it be to make themselves wealthier, even if all the side effects are not intentional?

There are examples and plenty of data that exist on the use of alternative therapies. The wonders of a lemon slice each day can facilitate anti-inflammation and weight loss. Turmeric and cinnamon have demonstrated effects on lowering blood glucose and improving insulin sensitivity. Alpha Lipoic Acid can be found in vegetable sources, with the highest content found in spinach, broccoli, tomatoes, peas, and Brussel sprouts to name a few. Alpha Lipoic Acid may sound like an intimidating name, but its benefits include positive effects and advantages against neurodegenerative diseases, diabetes, liver and heart disease, and myocardial and cerebral ischemia.

Dr. Frederick Robert Klenner practiced medicine in Reidsville, North Carolina years ago and believed the liver has a better chance of detoxifying the blood stream of poisons, toxins, viruses and bacteria if the plasma is saturated with Vitamin C. Linus Pauling was an American theoretical physical chemist who was inspired by Klenner and was a twice-honored Nobel Laureate. Pauling was known for work in chemical bonds and molecular structure which he applied to Vitamin C. His recommendation for high doses of vitamin C for the common cold is still recognized today. This is probably why many of us dash to the grocery store and place Vitamin C in our shopping carts. Interestingly, while we all know and have heard of Vitamin C, what type is better for you, 'L' or 'D'? The L-form is preferred and occurs naturally in the fruits and vegetables we eat. Vitamin C is a redox cofactor functioning in oxidative stress which has been proven to be associated with cellular damage and chronic illnesses. In fact, studies have demonstrated a significant association between smoking and elevated blood lead levels and daily supplementation with 1000mg of ascorbic acid has demonstrated a significant decrease in blood lead levels. Heavy metal toxicity is a term that is becoming increasingly popular and there are natural "chelators" which exist that can assist with this. The small amount of Vitamin C, recommended by the RDA (90mg) is enough to protect a person from gross disease, but not the amount to maintain good health. Higher than RDA intakes of vitamin C have been associated with several indices of lowered cardiovascular disease risk including increases in HDL, and decreases in LDL oxidation, blood pressure and cardiovascular mortality, yet continue to be underestimated and under researched.

Science has yet to grasp the magnificence of the human body. The complexity of the brain alone is "mind-blowing!" After all, what is a thought? An emotion? The number of feedback loops and chemical reactions occurring every second in the human body is no less than miraculous. You don't have to believe in miracles, but we can appreciate the beauty that surrounds us such as, but not limited to, the trees, the birds, and nature altogether. Or the fact that we live on a planet that is a miniscule part of a seemingly endless galaxy. At the very least, like the perspective that's all around us, as well as the fact that our journey here is temporary, maybe we can begin embracing the wonder of it all and become part of the solutions instead of the problem. We are the common factors of change!

The concept of health cost sharing is not new and dates to ancient times. So, what has changed, and why is there such a strong push to have everyone on healthcare insurance which mandates annual checkups...and those very checkups usually result in more medications? The champion effort to "Make America Healthy Again" is noble. But it must include informed consent freedom and flexibility for patients to seek help where they want to go, not where they are told, or even forced, to go. A presence of, or even an invitation to, holistic and natural therapies is an essential part of this progress to becoming healthier as a whole. Sharing the cost of healthcare lessens the financial burden that otherwise can lead to physical and emotional bankruptcy. Is insurance supposed to cover everything, or only what their limits and formularies allow? And why is one person being charged one price at one hospital, while another person pays a different price at the same facility?

Ethics and medicine should not discriminate. Dr. Martin Luther King stated in his "I Have A Dream" speech on August 28, 1963, as part of the March on Washington, that he envisioned a world where all men and women are created and treated equal; "We hold these truths to be self-evident, that all men are created equal, that they are endowed by their Creator with certain unalienable rights that among these are life, liberty, and the pursuit of happiness." Similarly, there is no room for racial inequality in the healthcare system. Furthermore, there is no room for financial discrimination—we help those who need help, period!

Patient advocacy is important as guidance is required to maneuver an ever-challenging healthcare system. Many patients do not even understand how to get started with an integrated approach to their health. We have choices in everyday life: to pray or not to pray, eat organic whole foods or choose foods that are nutrient-drained, and synthetically prepared, and laced with harmful chemicals infiltrated by chemicals and calories. Have you ever observed a person eating a "healthy salad," with a mound of blue cheese dressing? We can choose to take a half-dozen pharmaceutics each day when we're over the age of 50 (which seems to be the norm nowadays), or practice a healthy lifestyle that resonates with you. The choice is yours.

CareXchange is the north star of integrated health cost sharing, and we strive to drive financial solutions to our network. We will not stop, lay down, or quiet our voice until our community understands that the power of faith and health go hand in hand, while emphasizing education and awareness to successfully navigate the health journey. Is it possible there is a quantum effect that is spiritual, physical, and mental, all rolled into one that nobody can see? Some extra "life force" that somehow we know is there? Is that divinity in action? Lastly, we have attempted to capture overall health in the CareXchange formula^{TM} by considering the mathematical correlation between current state and incorporating changes in daily life in correlation with the God force as our compass.

Faith and love are so critical. The Bible specifically states in 1 Corinthians 13:13 the importance of faith, hope, and love—but the greatest of these is love. We may never know the answer to the infamous question of why some people live and others in the same situation, with the same disease, same age, same color, die. Our wish for you is that you understand the power of God's choreography and miraculous design in us, while understanding that you, too, have the power to educate yourself and take back control of your health using a different model—one that is not limited to drugs, but also blessed by wholesomeness and holistic wellness. There are miracles every day, and we wish the very best health for you, as well as the faith and love to change the world! God's speed! And, if you successfully challenged yourself in embarking on the Mystery hidden throughout these chapters, you have successfully unlocked the "Life Wellness Secret"!!

🔒LIFE WELLNESS SECRET UNLOCKED 🔒

"True health begins with awareness, is strengthened through empowerment and faith, flourishes in freedom and community, and blossoms through sharing, inspiration, and collective well-being."

AFTERWORD:
THE GREATER HEALING:
Together, We Rise

As you close this book, know this: you are not alone. Whether you're exploring health cost sharing for the first time or have walked this path for years, you're part of something deeply human—and deeply hopeful.

In a world often divided by fear, complexity, and rising costs, we see a different way: one built on community, compassion, and the timeless call to bear one another's burdens.

In a world where healthcare often feels cold, complicated, or out of reach, this ministry offers a different path: one rooted in people, not profit. In compassion, not bureaucracy. In shared burdens, not silent suffering. A hope that does not run dry. A love that lifts and lasts.

"Carry each other's burdens, and in this way you will fulfill the law of Christ."

—Galatians 6:2 (NIV)

In the valleys of illness and the peaks of recovery, this kind of sharing reminds us that God often heals not only through medicine, but through people—through kindness, prayer, and generosity. Is this a radical idea that we are each other's keepers? That love still matters. That generosity can triumph over scarcity. That faith can restore systems that feel broken. A hope that does not run dry. A love that lifts and lasts.

"They will know you by your love."

—John 13:35 (paraphrased)

The Life Wellness Collective isn't just about meeting medical needs. It's about reviving something ancient and beautiful: the belief that we're better together. That when we give, we receive. That the strength of a community is found in its willingness to love—no matter the cost. This community reflects the very best of what it means to be human—and the heart of a faith that still moves people to act with love. To the young and the old, the faithful and the curious: there's a place for you here. Every gift given, every prayer lifted, every burden shared tells a greater story—one of hope, healing, and belonging. Healing isn't just in medicine, it's in relationships. In showing up. In praying for someone you've never met. In giving from your heart, and trusting that others will do the same. So wherever you go from here, carry this truth: that faith still moves people, and people still move mountains.

"And let us not grow weary of doing good, for in due season
we will reap, if we do not give up."

—Galatians 6:9 (ESV)

Whether you've been walking with faith for years, are newly exploring, or simply believe in the power of human kindness, this journey is open to you. You are welcome here. Because we all share the same needs: to be seen, supported, and surrounded by a caring community. Even when the road feels long, we are sustained by a promise:

"Those who hope in the Lord will renew their strength.
They will soar on wings like eagles;
They will run and not grow weary,
They will walk and not be faint."

—Isaiah 40:31 (NIV)

This is just the beginning.

Let's keep building.
Keep caring.
Keep believing in each other—and maybe even in something greater.

To your health Journey,

The Authors

REFERENCES

Adams, M. (1967). Food Forensics: The Hidden Toxins Lurking in Your Food and How You Can Avoid Them For Lifelong Health. BenBella Books, Inc (2016).

Amin, K., Ortaliza, J., & Wager, E. (2025, October). Health Care Costs and Affordability. In D. Altman (Ed.), Health Policy 101. KFF. https://www.kff.org/health-policy-101-health-care-costs-and-affordability/

Batterson, M. (2024). A million little miracles: Rediscover the God who is bigger than big, closer than close, and gooder than good. Multnomah Chopra, D. (1989). Quantum healing:BExploring the frontiers of mind/body medicine. Bantam books.

Croskerry, P. (2010, March 23). To error is human–and let's not forget it. CMAJ, 182(5), 524. https://doi.org/10.1503/cmaj.100270

Emmerich, S.D., Fryar, C.D., Stierman, B., & Ogden, C.L. (2024). Obesity and severe prevalence in adults: United States, August 2021-August 2023 (NCHS Data Brief No. 508). National Center for Health Statistics. https://dx.doi.org/10.1562/cdc/150281

Hartweg, D.L., & Metcalfe, S.A. (2022, January). Orem's Self-Care Deficit Nursing Theory: Relevance and Need for Refinement. Nursing Science Quarterly, 35(1), 70-76. https://doi.org/10.1177/0894318421151369

Hawryluk, M. (2023, June 14). At least 1.7M Americans use health sharing arrangements, despite lack of protections. KFF Health News.https://kfhealthnews.org/news/article/health-sharing-arrangements- protection-risks/

Heathcott, J. (2003). The Black Panther Party and the fight against hunger in Oakland and beyond. Journal of Urban History.

Kaiser Family Foundation. 92025, October 28). ACA insurers are raising premiums by an estimated 26%, But most enrollees could see sharper increases in what they pay. Quick Take. https://www.kff.org/quick-take/ace-insurers-are-raising-premiums-by-an-estimated-26-but-most-enrollees-could-see-sharper-increases-in-what-they-pay/

Kaufman, E.L., Tress, J., & Sherry, D.D. (2017, May 1). Trends in Medicalization of Children with Amplified Musculoskeletal Pain Syndrome. Pain Medicine, 18(5), 825-831. https://doi.org/10.1093/pm/pnw188

King, M.L., Jr. (1963, August 28). I have a dream. The Avalon Project. https://avalon.law.yal.edu/20th_century/mlk10asp

Manning, B. (1996). The signature of Jesus. Multnomah.

Maslow, A.H. (1943). A theory of human motivation. Psychological Review, 50(4), 370-396.

Milbank Q. (2006, June). Health Planning in the United States and the Decline of Public Interest Policymaking. Milbank Quarterly, 84(2), 359-440. https://doi.org/10.1111/j.1468-0009.2006.00451.x

Millstone, D., Chen, C.Y., & Bauer, B. (2017, May 16). Complementary and integrative medicine in the management of headache. BMJ, 357, j1805. https://doi.org/10.1136/bmj.j1805

Molassiotis, A., & Chung, H.E. (2023). Regional Perspectives on Complementary and Alternative Medicine. https://pmc.ncbi.nlm.nih.gov/articles/PMC11633865/ National Center for Health Statistics. (2016). Use of complementary health approaches by U.S. Adults aged 18 and over: National Health Interview Survey, 2012 (NCHS Data Brief No.235).

Centers for Disease Control and Prevention.
https://www.cdc.gov/nchs/data/databrief/db235.pdf

Roosevelt, T. (1910, April 23). Citizenship in a republic. In J. Smith (Ed.), Speeches that changed the world (pp. 45-50). Penguin Books.

Schultz, H. (2016, December 2). My interview with Starbucks CEO Howard Schultz. Carmine Gallo.

Shaw, G.B. (1949). Back to Methuselah. In Selected plays with prefaces (Vol. 2, p. 7). Dodd, Mead.

Shelly, M. (1823) Personal Conversations with Mary Shelly.

Swerdlow, R.H. (2014). British Journal of Pharmacology, Vol. 171, pages 1854-1869.

Taddei, A. (2012). The 5 biological laws and Dr. Hamer's new medicine. (Kindle ed.). Amazon Digital Services LLC.

Thoreau, H.D. (1854). Walden UnitedHealth Group. (2017). UnitedHealthcare Consumer Sentiment Survey. UnitedHealth Group.

26 U.S.C. & 5000A (d) (2). (2010). Legal information Institute. https://www.law.cornell.edu/definitions/uscode.php

U.S. Department of Health and Human Services. (2025). Make America Healthy Again (MAHA). https://www.hhs.gov/maha/index.html

Wachowski, L., & Wachowski, L. (Directors) (1999). The Matrix [Film]. Warner Bros.; Village Roadshow Pictures; Groucho Film Partnership.

ABOUT THE AUTHORS

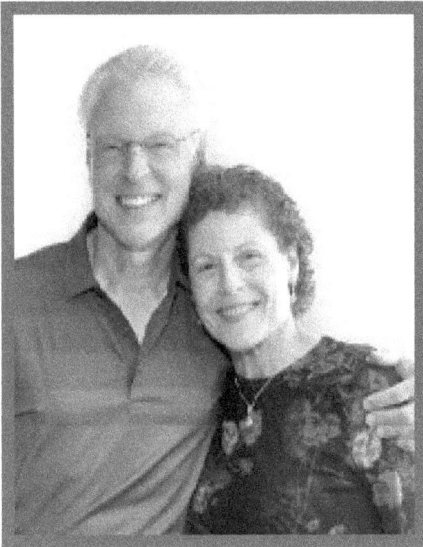

Dr. David M. Shearer, MD and Dorothy M. Shearer, MS, RN, are a compassionate team with decades of combined experience in healthcare and healing. Together, they have dedicated their lives to guiding others toward health and wholeness through an integrative approach that honors both the wisdom of modern medicine and the healing power of natural holistic practices. A dynamic duo, both within their marriage and professional life, David and Dorothy believe in addressing the whole person—body, mind, and spirit—while encouraging food as medicine, mindful living, and faith-centered wellness. Their philosophy is rooted in compassion and empowerment, inviting people to look beyond prescriptions and quick fixes to discover the sustaining benefits of whole foods, natural remedies, and a balanced lifestyle. In both their professional practice and daily lives, they embody the principles they teach, "walking the walk" with open hearts and open minds. Their shared mission is to help others find awareness, strength, and hope on the journey to health. As authors of The Life Wellness Collective and creators of CareXchange, David and Dorothy Shearer bring not only their clinical expertise but also their humanity, faith, and lived experience, offering readers a roadmap to healing that is both practical and deeply personal. Their message is simple yet profound: true wellness begins when we combine knowledge with compassion and live with intention.

www.ingramcontent.com/pod-product-compliance
Lightning Source LLC
Chambersburg PA
CBHW060233030426
42335CB00014B/1435